10/82

OPHTHALMIC SURFACING

for Plastic and Glass Lenses

ISBN-0-87873-041-9

Library of Congress Catalog Card Number:81-84855

Published by The Professional Press, Inc.
101 East Ontario Street, Chicago, Illinois 60611

Printed in the U.S.A.

OPHTHALMIC SURFACING
for Plastic and Glass Lenses

by
Richard J. Mancusi

The Professional Press, Inc.
Chicago, Illinois

TABLE OF CONTENTS

APPENDIX I

APPENDIX II

APPENDIX III

FIGURES

INTRODUCTION

The purpose of this text is to compile and update basic ophthalmic laboratory procedures. For ease of use, the material has been divided into three sections. The first section covers the basic surface shop in a step-by-step manner. The second section discusses procedures that are more complex or less often used. The third section contains a collection of charts for easy reference.

What little has been written about plastic lens fabrication stresses the differences between it and glass lens fabrication. This has given the entire process an unnecessary reputation as being difficult. The main thrust of this text is plastic lenses and their similarity to glass lenses. Although it is thoroughly covered, glass lens fabrication is treated as an adjunct to plastic lens fabrication. It is hoped that this substantial change in the manner these topics are covered will remove some of the stigma created by people who stressed the problems encountered with plastic that were not generally associated with glass.

It is highly unlikely that everyone will agree that every idea or procedure in this book is totally correct. Out of necessity, procedures vary from lab to lab due to equipment, conditions, or manpower. No individual's methods or manufacturer's machinery has been intentionally slighted. The specifics of a method or machine's operations are best left to the expertise of the manufacturer's manual.

To facilitate your reading, a prerequisite knowledge of basic optics is suggested. The following books may be useful as background reading:

J. L. Cockrum, *Optician Students Manual,* Austin, Tex.; University of Texas at Austin, 1975.

John B. Epting and Frank C. Morgret, Jr., *Ophthalmic Mechanics and Dispensing,* Radnor, Penn.: Chilton Book Company, 1964.

Meredith W. Morgan, *The Optics of Ophthalmic Lenses,* Chicago: Professional Press, 1978.

OPHTHALMIC SURFACING

for Plastic and Glass Lenses

SECTION I

The Basic Surface Shop

Chapter 1.
Selecting the Lens

Finished Lens

Finished lenses must be your paramount thought when determining the lens blank needs of a single-vision prescription. Using finished lenses rather than semifinished lenses will do the following:
1. Speed the prescription through the shop.
2. Save unnecessary wear on the surface shop machinery.
3. Save the cost of surface shop fabricating materials.
4. Reduce by one-half the possibility of a lens spoilage.
5. Reduce the surface shop worker hours.

Keep an up-to-date list of your stock range and readily available finished lenses. Extended delays caused by special orders of finished lenses negate their use.

The key to using finished lenses lies in the accurate determination of cutout. The only sure way to see if the lens will cut out is to spot and mark it up in the finish shop. It would be a waste of the finish shop's time and make lens pulling much too big a project to check each prescription for cutout in this manner. That is why a quicker method must be used.

First, measure the frame using the boxing system (see Figure I). Measure from the right eye nasal box to the left eye temporal box. This is the distance between the left and right eye geometric centers and is referred to as the **frame size** or **frame PD**.

The total decentration is the difference between this measurement and the patient's PD. Do not divide the total decentration by two to obtain the decentration per eye. For every millimeter the lens is decentered, 2mm of lens blank is used. By using the total decentration rather than the decentration per eye, this factor is compensated for.

The smallest finished lens able to be used with the prescription is obtained by adding the total decentration to the longest, generally diagonal, measurement of the eye. As an example, say the frame measures 72mm and the patient's PD is 64mm. The total decentration is 72 - 64, or 8mm. If the longest measurement of the eye is 56mm, the smallest usable lens is 56 + 8, or 64mm. If decentration per eye rather than PD is given on the prescription, simply double the per-eye decentration to obtain the total decentration, and proceed as explained above.

Occasionally the optical center (OC) of the finished lens may not be at the geometric center of the blank. Depending on the axis of the prescription, this may or may not assist in obtaining the decentration. This system for selecting finished lens blank size is not infallible, but it is rapid and relatively accurate.

Semifinished Lens

If after using this method you find that finished lenses do not fulfill your prescription requirements, a semifinished lens must be used.

Determining Blank Size

Single Vision
Since we can locate the optical center anywhere on a semifinished lens, selecting the blank diameter becomes simple. Basically all you need is enough lens diameter to fill the eye size at its longest diameter. Realistically, allow yourself 4mm of "extra" lens. This is only 2mm on either side of the finished lens. In this area you must absorb chips, bevel, and slightly mislocated optical centers.

Be aware of how large your lens blanks actually are. Do your 65mm lenses measure 65mm, or do they really measure 64mm? Also consider the optical soundness of the blank all the way to its periphery. These factors generally reduce most lens blanks by 1mm. Say, for example, the longest measurement of the frame eye is 58mm. Allowing approximately 2mm for chips, bevel, and so forth, this expands the needed diameter to 60mm. Allowing a 1mm reduction in lens blank diameter, you can see that a 60mm lens will not be large enough, a 62mm lens would just make it, and a 65mm lens would be comfortable. The use of a larger lens blank would be a foolish waste of money.

Executive Style
The selection of multifocal lens blanks depends on the style of multifocal. The executive-style blank size selection is greatly affected by the method of fabrication. If the optical center is to be decentered by grinding prism, you need only enough lens diameter to fill the eye size. The blank size should be selected as you would a semifinished single-vision blank. The inability to

control both the distance and near optical centers encourages some labs to grind without prism. You would then make a lens similar to a finished single-vision blank, with blank size selected accordingly.

The only factor that separates the executive-style multifocal from the single vision is the need to consider the segment (seg) height. Instead of simply considering how the blank is moving in and out, you must also consider the blank movement up and down. Establish how far below center the seg line is by dividing the B measurement of the lens blank by two and subtracting the height of the seg line. Say the B measurement of the blank is 60mm. The height of the seg line is 26mm. 60 ÷ 2 = 30; 30 − 26 = 4. The seg line is 4mm below the geometric center of the blank (Figure 2).

To find out how much the blank must be moved, it is necessary to approximate the finished layout. This is calculated in exactly the same way as the seg line drop on the blank. Divide the B measurement of the frame by two and calculate the difference between that measurement and the requested seg height. We will not necessarily be able to subtract the seg height from ½B, because it is possible to have a seg height above center. Say the B measurement of the frame is 40mm. The requested seg height is 22mm. 40 ÷ 2 = 20; 22 − 20 = 2. This would be 2mm above—not 2mm below—center (Figure 3).

To finish the blank size selection, combine the two examples. The first example shows that the seg line is 4mm below, while the second example shows that you need 2mm above. The blank seg line will need to move 6mm with respect to the geometric center of the blank. Remember that with every 1mm of movement, 2mm of lens is needed. We therefore use 12mm of blank. Add this 12mm to the 40mm B measurement of the frame and obtain 52mm. Adding the 2mm of chip-bevel tolerance nets a minimum blank B dimension of 54mm. You are taking what you already used through the horizontal and applying it through the vertical meridian.

Flat Top Multifocal and Other Styles

Flat top multifocal blank size selection is a combination of finished single-vision and executive procedures. A finished single-vision lens has something in it that is nonmovable but must be located exactly in the finished product—the optical center. The segment in a flat top bifocal is precisely the same. Finding out where the segment lies in the blank and then combining this knowledge with where it must be in the finished product will determine the necessary blank size.

The vertical placement of the top of the seg line is determined exactly as with the executive: ½B − seg line height. To determine horizontal placement, divide the A measurement of the blank by two. Subtract this from the measurement taken from the temporal side of the blank to the center of the seg on the same line the A measurement of the blank was taken. As an example, the A measurement of the blank in Figure 4 is 64mm. The center of the seg is 37mm in from the temporal edge of the lens. 64 ÷ 2 = 32; 37 − 32 = 5. The seg is set in 5mm from the geometric center of the lens blank.

Now that you can establish seg placement, you are ready to calculate a blank size. Since the seg is near point, you must work with the near PD. Subtract the near PD from the frame size or frame PD. Obtain the near

18787.81
7563.

W - 18787.81
M - 7.563.76
CROSS - 26.351.57

4053.46
885.62

FEDERAL TAX 4.939.08

decentration per eye by diving by two. This is the amount the seg must be moved in. But since the seg is already decentered in some, the blank will only be moving the difference between the seg and needed decentration. The amount the blank—not the seg—is moved must be doubled and treated exactly like a finished single-vision lens to determine the horizontal blank size.

The vertical movement is figured as you did with executives. Assume frame size 74mm, near PD 60mm, seg height 14mm, B measurement 40mm, seg placement 5 in 4 down, longest frame eye measurement 56mm. $74 - 60 = 14 \div 2 = 7$ in. Since the seg is already in 5mm, the blank needs to move 2mm horizontally. $40 \div 2 = 20 - 14 = 6$ down. Since the seg is already down 4mm, the seg must only move 2mm vertically. Four millimeters of lens blank is used horizontally and 4mm vertically, a total of 8mm. $56 + 8 = 64$mm. Adding the 2mm of tolerance, a 66mm blank is the smallest lens blank able to fabricate this prescription. All you have done is figured a finished single-vision lens horizontally and vertically, taking into account the placement of a nonmovable point—the seg.

Determining blank size of most other seg styles involves a combination of procedures already shown. A round seg, for example, is a flat top with the ability to expand its blank size by rotating the segment in. By combining these methods you should be able to find a workable method for the blank size selection of any style of multifocal.

Selecting Base Curve

After determining the semifinished blank size, the selection of base curve remains. It is very doubtful that you could find two lens manufacturers or major optical laboratories that could agree on a base curve chart. There is not any one correct method. With this in mind, we will outline a system to be used as a starting point toward the development of a workable system for you. Your system must be based on the manufacturer and base curves you use. For the sake of simplicity we will use the even base curves of plano, 2, 4, 6, 8, 10, and 12.

-8.00 to -12.00D . . .	pl base
-5.00 to -9.00D . . .	2 base
-1.50 to -6.00D . . .	4 base
Pl to -2.00D . . .	6 base
Pl to $+2.00$D . . .	6 base
$+1.50$ to $+6.00$D . . .	8 base
$+5.00$ to $+9.00$D . . .	10 base
$+8.00$ to $+11.00$D . . .	12 base

This is considered a fairly liberal chart that extends the range of the base curve about as far as you would want. All charts are based on what the resultant inside curve will be. A plano lens should have approximately a -6.00D inside curve. The higher you go in minus, the further the inside curve may deviate from -6.00 in the minus direction. The higher you go in plus, the further the inside curve may deviate from -6.00 in the plus direction. In other words, having inside curves of −8.00, −10.00, or −12.00D in higher minus is acceptable, while having inside curves of −5.00, −3.00, or −1.00D in higher plus is acceptable.

Factors in Selection

To this point we have only discussed simple spherical powers. When a cylinder is added, it may become necessary to adjust your selection. Again we are looking at the inside curve we are creating. A −2.00 on a 6 base creates an acceptable −8.00 inside curve. What if the prescription is −2.00 combined with a −5.00 cylinder? The inside curve becomes an unacceptable −8.00/−13.00. The prescription should be put on either 4 or 2 base, giving you inside curves of −6.00/−11.00 or −4.00/−9.00, respectively.

Another factor that may cause you to adjust your selection is the power of the other eye. If one eye is a +1.75 sphere, you would probably select a 6 base lens, giving you a −4.25 inside curve. If the other eye is a +2.25, you would probably select an 8 base lens, giving you a −5.75 inside curve. Independently, each selection is satisfactory. Considering both eyes of the prescription, the base curve selections are unacceptable. For optical soundness and to increase patient acceptance, it is important that the inside curves be as similar as is reasonably possible. In this case, there is a 1.50D difference in inside curves when there is only a 0.50D difference in power. This can be rectified by putting both lenses on the same base curve. The best selection would probably be 8 base. However, depending on the style of frame, 6 base may be the best selection.

This brings up another factor that may affect your selection—the frame. Do not make fabricating or mounting problems for the finish shop. A −2.00 −1.00 can be put on a 6 base blank. However, if the lens is going into a large rimless or metal frame, 4 base would be a better selection. This flatter base curve will give you a flatter inside curve and thus less frame bending. This will reduce the odds of breaking the frame while increasing the odds of a good-looking and well-fitting mounting. Even some zyl frames have a tendency to pop lenses when they have too steep an inside or outside curve. At the other extreme, the very small half-eyes will look better if you lean toward using a slightly flatter base curve.

Another reason to flatten the base curve is excessive prism. A plano lens with 8.00D of prism is much easier to fabricate and better looking on 4 base rather than 6 base.

The last factor we will discuss that may affect your blank selection is the blank manufacturer. Manufacturers vary substantially on blank parameters. Center thickness, edge thickness, and rough inside curve greatly influence the finished inside curve range possible on the blank. For example, one manufacturer uses a −10.00 rough inside curve on its 6 base blanks. It would be a relatively simple task to put a finished −12.00 inside curve on its lens blank. Another lens manufacturer uses a −6.00 rough inside curve on its 6 base blanks. Their blank would have to be very thick (which it is not) to change that −6.00 to a −12.00.

Considering all the factors that affect the selection of base curve, it is obviously impossible for any one chart to be correct all the time. If you start with the basic chart and make your adjustments based on what you just read, you cannot be far off. When you run into a plus power beyond the chart, it will generally be in the form of an aspheric lens. Follow the manufacturer's suggestion for your base curve selection. Minus beyond the chart can be handled in any number of ways. In plastic lenses the solution usually is a shift to another style (double concave, myodisc, or minus lenticular). In glass lenses one of those forms or a glass of heavier density, such as highlight, may be used.

Chapter 2.
Figuring the Shop Slip

The cost of layout computers is down to the point where it would be foolish to perform layout by hand. However, do not be led astray. A computer is an excellent tool, but, like any tool, it works only as well as the individual using it allows. Are your plus lenses coming out too thick? Check the printout—was that ED really 54, or was it actually 52? Programmers will tell you: garbage in, garbage out. In other words, a computer computes based on the information you give it. If you give it inaccurate information, do not expect good-looking lenses. The computer is an aid, a vital ally, but it is not perfect.

I doubt that there are two computers programmed alike. There are many differences between computer programs, and computers differ on two basic ideas. (1) Blocking of multifocals: Some computers figure the necessary prism for on-center blocking, while the others figure for traditional blocking. (2) Prism on single vision: Some computers consider the size blank you are using and grind only the amount of prism necessary after the blank has been decentered as far as possible. The other method grinds the total decentration. Which is the correct method? There is not one correct method, but rather a method that you find more comfortable.

Each programmer has his own ideas, not necessarily coinciding with yours. Do not be afraid to edit the computer slip. I know one highly automated lab with a very sophisticated computer. Because the employees are encouraged to do just what the computer prints out without editing, some very interesting glasses occasionally are fabricated. This computer is programmed to do all single-vision lenses, beyond − 19.00D in the myodic form. Guess what happened when a prescription came in with a − 19.00 OD and a − 19.25 OS? That's right, one myodisc and one not. It actually got all the way through the shop and to the account. While this is obviously an extreme, the point stands. For top-quality, fast work you cannot beat the *team* effort of you and the computer.

Understand the Computer—Lens Power

It is a good idea to know how the computer arrives at its conclusions. The power of the lens is basically the difference between its inside and outside curves. The thickness and index of refraction are the major factors that would alter this rule of thumb.

Thickness does not significantly affect the power until approximately 4.0mm at the optical center. Considering regular crown glass, the power of a minus lens would be only the combination of the curves; e.g., a lens having a + 6.50 base curve with a − 7.50 inside curve would have a net power of − 1.00. A cylindrical prescription is created by adding a cross curve to the inside of the lens. For example, a lens having a + 6.50 base curve with a − 7.50/ − 8.00 inside curve would have a net power of − 1.00 − 0.50. It is just that simple as long as the thickness remains below 4.0mm at the optical center.

If you change lens materials from crown to 1.7 index highlight, it is necessary to make a compensation. By multiplying the requested prescription power by 0.76, you will obtain the compensated power at the highlight index. For example, multiplying the requested prescription power of − 6.00 by 0.76, you obtain the compensated power of − 4.56. This power combined with the front curve will give you the needed inside curve. A 4.50 base highlight lens used to grind a − 6.00 sphere will require a 9.06 inside curve: 4.50 + 4.56 = 9.06. The cylindrical amount must also be compensated for with the same 0.76 factor.

If the lens material is plastic, the same idea is used, but with a different multiplication factor. With plastic, multiply the requested prescription power by 1.065. The only procedural difference may come with the cylindrical value. Since most labs use separate tools for plastic lenses, it is possible to build the cylindrical compensation into the tool. If this is your situation, add the uncompensated requested cylinder onto the compensated inside sphere curve to obtain the needed inside cross curve. It does not matter whether you compensate at layout or with your tools. The important thing is to compensate once and only once.

Thickness and Inside Curve

If the finished lens is to be over approximately 4.0mm at the optical center, the inside curve must be compensated. The thicker the lens, the steeper the inside curve must be. There are charts available that show the approximate increase in inside curve as related to the thickness. To obtain a true appreciation of what the computer does, or what you should do to obtain the correct answer, we must look at the formula for calculating inside curve:

$$I_c = O_c - P + \frac{T}{\mu}(O_c)^2$$

That is, the inside curve equals the outside curve minus the requested power plus the thickness at the optical center in meters divided by the index of refraction times the outside curve squared. Say the outside, or base, curve is +10.50. The requested power is +8.50. The thickness is 7.8mm and the index of refraction is 1.523. What is the needed inside curve?

$$I_c = 10.50 - 8.50 + \frac{0.0078}{1.523}(10.50)^2$$

$$I_c = 2.56$$

Determining Thickness

Now you know how to obtain the needed inside curve for any lens material or index at any thickness. The next problem is how to determine the needed thickness. Again, we have charts and the formula used to develop the charts:

$$T = R - \sqrt{R^2 - \left(\frac{D}{2}\right)^2}$$

The thickness equals the radius of curvature in millimeters minus the square root of the radius of curvature squared minus one-half the longest diameter of the finished lens squared. Now, how thick should a +5.00D lens 50mm in diameter be?

$$T = 104.6 \sqrt{(104.6)^2 - \left(\frac{50}{2}\right)^2}$$

$$T = 3.03$$

The next logical question is how do you obtain the radius of curvature needed for the thickness formula. The formula for obtaining the radius of curvature follows.

$$R = \frac{\mu - 1}{P}$$

The radius of curvature in meters equals the index of refraction minus one divided by the power in diopters.

What would be the radius of curvature of a 5.00D lens? Traditionally, tools are calculated on 1.530 index.

$$R = \frac{1.530 - 1}{5}$$

$$R = 0.106$$

Since the thickness formula requires the radius of curvature in millimeters, move the decimal point three places to the right. The answer is therefore 106.

There are two other factors that affect the thickness of a lens: the movement of the optical center by decentration or prism, and the adjustment to a usable thickness of the knife edge strap thickness created by the thickness formula. The diameter of the finished lens in the thickness formula should be increased by the amount of decentration. For example, a 50mm lens decentered 2mm should be considered to have a 54mm diameter. If the optical center is to be moved by prism, do not consider the decentration. Instead, a good rule of thumb is to add 0.5mm of thickness for every 1.00D of prism to the final thickness.

Add the amount of desired strap thickness onto the needed center thickness. If after all the adjustments you find the center thickness to be, say, 5.0, add to it the strap thickness you want. 5.0 + 1.8 = 6.8, that is, a 5.0 center thickness at a knife edge plus a 1.8 strap thickness equals a 6.8 center thickness.

Calculating Prism

The next thing to consider is how you calculate the necessary prism. The formula is the following:

$$\Delta = \frac{P \times D}{10}$$

The prism equals the power of the lens times the amount of decentration divided by ten. (Find the amount of decentration exactly as you did when selecting finished single-vision blanks.) How much prism is necessary, then, to decenter the optical center 5mm on a 4.00D lens?

$$\Delta = \frac{4 \times 5}{10}$$

$$\Delta = 2.0$$

This formula gives you the ability to locate the optical center any place you want on the lens blank. When a 65mm finished lens will not cut out, it is very possible that a 65mm semifinished lens will. With the finished lens it is necessary to physically move the entire lens to obtain the decentration. With the semifinished lens, however, the blank can stay on center, because the optical center in the blank has been decentered by prism. When grinding prism for decentration, we are moving the optical center through the 180-degree meridian. Therefore, it is necessary to use the power running through the 180-degree meridian in the formula.

A sphere has the same power running through all of its meridians and thus presents no problem. A cylinder, however, does not maintain the same power in all its meridians. The cylindrical part of a prescription is not a power, but rather a difference in power between the meridians. What you need to ascertain is how much the difference will affect the sphere power at 180 degrees. Again, there are charts and the following formula:

$$P = C \times \sin^2 A$$

The difference power equals the amount of cylinder times the sine squared of the angle of the cylinder. In the prescription $-1.00\ -3.00 \times 30$, how much will the cylinder power affect the sphere power through the 180-degree meridian?

$$P = -3 \times \sin^2 30$$

$$P = -0.75$$

The total power through the 180-degree meridian is the amount of the sphere power combined with the effect of the cylinder. For example, $-1.00 + (-0.75) = -1.75$. The -1.75 is the power that would be used in the prism formula to obtain the necessary prism through the 180-degree meridian.

The direction or base of the prism is based on whether the power is plus or minus through the meridian of the prism. An easy way to remember which way to go is that a minus lens has a negative or opposite sign in front of the amount of power. Therefore, if you wish to move the optical center in, the prism base must be in the opposite direction, out. Whichever direction you wish to move the optical center, the base of the prism must be opposite on a minus lens. With a plus lens the prism base is the same direction as the direction of optical center movement.

How much prism is necessary to decenter the optical center in 5mm on the prescription $-2.25\ -.75 \times 45$?

$$P = C \times \sin^2 A$$

$$P = -0.75 \times \sin^2 45$$

$$P = -0.375$$

$-2.25 + (-0.375) = -2.625$, the power through the 180-degree meridian.

$$\Delta = \frac{P \times D}{10}$$

$$\Delta = \frac{-2.625 \times 5}{10}$$

$$\Delta = -1.31$$

The minus sign on the amount of prism tells you that it will run the opposite direction. Therefore, to move the optical center in 5mm on the prescription $-2.25 -0.75 \times 45$, it is necessary to grind 1.30D of prism base out.

A prescription may require prism in more than one meridian. It may ask for prism base up or down and prism base in or out. Or a prescription may ask for prism in only one meridian, but you also calculate the need for prism to move the optical center. If the two prisms lie in the same meridian, you may simply combine them. Say the prescription asks for 2Δ out, and you calculate 1Δ out for decentration; the result is 3Δ out. The prescription asks for 2Δ out, and you calculate 3Δ in for decentration; the result is 1Δ in. If the prisms lie in two different meridians, 2Δ up and 2Δ in, a chart or formula must be used:

$$R = \sqrt{P_1{}^2 + P_2{}^2}$$

The resultant prism equals the square root of the first prism squared plus the second prism squared. Find the resultant prism: 2Δ up combined with 2Δ in.

$$R = \sqrt{(2)^2 + (2)^2}$$

$$R = 2.8\Delta$$

The 2.8Δ is the amount of prism. Now using another formula you must find the direction or base of the prism.

$$\tan A = \frac{P_1}{P_2}$$

The tangent of the angle is equal to the prism up or down divided by the prism in or out.

$$\tan A = \frac{2}{2}$$
$$A = 45°$$

This 45 degrees is the prism axis deviation from the 180-degree line.

Whether you are working with a right or left eye will determine the actual axis. If in this example the 2Δ up and 2Δ in were in a right eye, the resultant axis would be 45 degrees. If it were in a left eye, the axis would be 135 degrees. Using a 180 degree protractor, we would refer to these results as 45 degrees base up and in and 135 degrees base up and in. If the prism were running down and in, the answers would be 135 degrees base down and in on the right eye and 45 degrees base down and in on the left eye. A 360-degree protractor can simplify the axis designation. The following chart compares the two protractor designations. See also Figures 5 and 6.

EYE	180°	360°
Right	45° up and in	45°
Left	135° up and in	135°
Right	135° down and in	315°
Left	45° down and in	225°

You now have enough information to lay out most single-vision prescriptions. Multifocals other than executives generally do not have the distance optical center decentered by using prism. They should be treated like a single-vision lens that is not having prism for decentration ground on it. In other words, the amount the blank is to be decentered should be added to the finished blank size for use in the thickness formula. Prism that must be ground on a multifocal is calculated the same as in single vision.

Multifocals ground using the on-center blocking system must have resultant or compound prism ground to move the distance optical center from the geometric center of the blank to its proper location by the segment. To calculate the proper location of the distance optical center with regard to the segment, you must consider both the PD and the frame B dimension. Horizontally the optical center must be decentered out from the center of the segment the difference between the distance and near PDs on a per-eye basis. Vertically the optical center should lie in the middle of the frame, or at one-half B. The exception to the vertical point would be if one-half B lies closer than 2mm from the seg line, or in the segment itself. If the distance optical center is ground too close to the seg line, a poor neutralization will result. If the lens is to be blocked any place other than those calculations, as in on-center blocking, compound prism must be ground to move the optical center to where it belongs.

Recommendations

This completes a basic look at hand layout. Whether you choose to use charts or the formulas, be careful. Many a prescription has been laid out wrong by someone who ran their finger down the wrong column of a chart. The math in the formulas is very simple, but there are too many places to make a mistake. If you wish to use the formulas, I highly recommend a twenty-dollar investment in a calculator. Even that small amount should give you a calculator that will fly through the formulas. Realistically, an inexpensive layout computer is the best way to go, considering the accuracy and time savings it offers.

Chapter 3.
Lens Markup

Edit the computer slip carefully, changing the things necessary to fit your system.

Factors to Consider

Check the lens carefully for scratches, pits, and straightness and width of the seg line. Follow the computer slip's parameters carefully, as any deviation at this point will result in substantial problems. Whether you use a computer or lay out by hand, the important data should be circled or highlighted to avoid confusion.

Consider what information the various areas of the surface shop require, and mark that information so that it may be seen easily. At the marker you need to know the axis of the cylinder, axis of the prism, and, in the case of multifocals, decentration with respect to the segment. The generator operator needs to know the curves to be cut, the amount of prism needed, and either the amount of lens material to be removed (take off) or the base curve, depending on the type of generator. The cylinder machine operators need to know the tool curve, amount of prism, and need for calipering. Although some labs caliper all lenses, it should be adequate to caliper only the lenses with 0.50D or less running through any meridian. Put a C (for caliper) on the shop slip of the lenses to be calipered. Labs generally use a red grease pencil to circle these needed facts.

Markup

After the shop slip has been edited, you are ready to mark up the lenses. Single-vision lenses are generally marked by hand on a protractor. (See Figure 7.) Using either a white grease pencil or marking ink pen, draw a straight line across the lens to indicate that the lens has cylinder on it. If the lens also has prism, turn the line to the cylindrical axis and then score another line through the prism axis. Indicate the base of the prism by an arrowhead on the prism axis line. This is where you will line up the generator prism ring (that is, assuming your prism rings are marked at their apex rather than base). If your prism rings are marked at their base, the arrowhead must be put at the opposite end of the prism axis line.

If the lens is a sphere, no lines are necessary unless the lens requires prism. In the case of a sphere with prism, draw a line through 90 degrees and a second line for the prism at the prism axis. If a lens chips on the generator, it is usually through the horizontal, not vertical axis. Most single-vision prism is for PD and therefore runs through the 180-degree meridian. By using two 90-degree opposed lines on spheres, any generator chips will reduce the blank size through the B dimension rather than the A dimension. Since most frames are larger through the A than B dimension, this procedure could save a possible lens spoilage.

Multifocals are marked similarly. (See Figure 8.) Most labs use a marking machine that backlights and magnifies the lens. A protractor will work but is perhaps slightly slower or less accurate. Using either method, the first step is to locate the segment down and in according to the layout slip. Once this is accomplished, the cylinder and prism axis lines can be marked. Spherical multifocals should be marked at axis 90 degrees for the same reason as the single vision lens. Once you have marked the cylinder and prism axis lines on either the single vision or multifocal lens, put an R or L on the lens to avoid right and left lens mix-ups. You are now ready to proceed to precoating.

Chapter 4.
Precoat

There are many different types of precoat in liquid, brush-on, and spray form. Many labs mix more than one type to obtain the desired result. Your selection should be based on the strength of hold desired, laboratory humidity, ventilation, and background color desired. With the variety available you should have no trouble finding a suitable precoat at a reasonable price.

Another type of precoat is the 3M-Armorlite tape system. This is basically a wide, heat-resistant tape that is sticky on both sides. It is applied with a special vacuum machine directly to the lens surface. All these methods are good and deserve your experimentation.

Precoat Functions

Precoat or tape serves three functions in the glass surface shop. The first function is protection. During processing the finished side of the lens must be protected. The second function is adhesion. The precoat or tape acts as an aid in the adhesion of the alloy and block to the lens. The third function is providing a colored background to aid lens inspection during fabrication.

In the plastic shop, heat is one of the biggest problems. In addition to the three glass precoat functions, plastic precoat or tape is designed to provide the fourth function, a heat shield. Without a proper heat shield, the surface of a plastic lens could be destroyed during the blocking process.

Chapter 5.
Blocking

Temperature—Plastic Lens

The alloy used for blocking plastic lenses has a melting temperature of 117°F. The alloy must be molten and flow easily while staying as close to 117°F. as possible. Most blockers have two thermostats: one for the pot, to keep the alloy molten, and one for the throat, to help the alloy flow out of the blocker. Use both thermostats together to help maintain the lowest possible temperature; i.e., do not turn the pot temperature up when the alloy is molten in the pot but does not flow well—the problem is in the throat temperature.

Use a thermometer to check both temperatures. If the temperature is over 125°F. you have serious problems:

1. The two thermostats are not balanced properly.
2. The alloy lines are clogged with contaminated alloy which requires more heat to become molten. This is caused by not keeping the reclaim tank clean enough and running the blocker too low on alloy. This contaminated alloy will generally float on the alloy, so if you keep the alloy level up the lines will not get clogged.
3. If your blocker uses air line feed, the air pressure is too low.
4. If you use a hand pump blocker, the diaphragm probably has a hole in it.

Between the precoat and blocker temperature, you can see we go to great lengths to keep the heat to a minimum. Besides this, most labs run either a water ring to the blocker or chill the blocks; some labs do both. If you choose to chill the blocks, make sure that you do not get an excessive amount of condensation on the block prior to blocking. This water could create a loose block or even mark the lens surface.

Blocks

The argument for using the smallest possible block is obvious. The smaller the block, the less heat-creating alloy is necessary to attach it to the lens. The problem with plastic lenses is that they are far less rigid than glass. Therefore, the argument is raised that we need a larger, more rigid backing to assure even surface quality. This larger backing surface can be accomplished in either of two ways: (1) Using the standard Coburn glass blocks with special blocking molds. These molds extend the alloy out past the block in various amounts, depending on the mold selected. (2) Using Coburn or other manufacturers' special plastic lens blocks. Varying in size, the blocks themselves provide the different backing. I have seen both of these systems work extremely well. I have also been very impressed with the quality of work obtained by using the standard Coburn glass block with no additional backing. This is a very individual selection based on the type of work you are doing, type of machinery, personnel, and your computer.

Procedure—Plastic Lens

Now you are ready to block. Select and chill blocks with base curves as similar to the lenses as possible. The more similar the base curves, the less alloy used. This will keep the heat buildup to a minimum, and the lenses will be ready for generating sooner.

Place the chilled block into the appropriate water ring or mold body, depending on the system you are using. Align this combination on the blocker with the block's axis horizontal and the blocker spout through the block. With the precoated surface toward the block, align the len's axis and center lines with the block's axis and center marks. In the case of a single vision lens you may have an axis line but no center line. Then simply center the lens on the block, keeping the lens's axis line horizontal to the block's axis line (Figure 9).

The next step is to fill the mold with alloy. Fill the mold completely and rapidly. Most blocking systems have some sort of alloy release port in case of mold overfill; usually a cut in the block or mold. Do not rely on this. With a little practice the blocker can be controlled to fill without overfilling. The danger in overfilling is that prism can be induced when alloy is allowed to seep out beyond the intended limits.

With some systems the generator rings go directly on the lens. The angle of the block will not affect the prism, but if alloy seeps out onto the area where the generator ring will rest, prism will be induced. In other systems the generator rings go directly on the block. If the segment of the lens or alloy tips the block even slightly, prism will result.

After the mold is filled, remove the blocked lens from it and either allow it to cool gradually at room temperature or rechill it for a short time. You have a temperature problem if the alloy is not cooling rapidly enough after filling for you to immediately be able to separate the blocked lens from the mold. Either the alloy is too warm, or the blocks or water ring are not being chilled adequately. If a lens separates from the block and alloy when everything is cool and the alloy hard, there is one of two problems. Either moisture on the surface of the overchilled block was not wiped off, or the lens was cooled too rapidly after blocking. After the alloy has hardened and everything is to room temperature, the lens may be generated. The waiting time could run up to one-half hour, depending on how well you controlled the temperature.

Procedure—Glass

In the glass surface shop the same procedures apply, but with far less emphasis on heat problems. Although the alloy used in blocking melts at 158°F., the chance of heat damaging the surface of a glass lens is slight. This does not mean that alloy temperatures should not be monitored. Excessively high temperatures can adversely affect a precoat's adhesion and the alloy setup time. If the lens is removed from the blocking ring before the alloy is adequately set up, a lens that is off axis or has prism induced may result. If the alloy temperature is properly monitored, it is totally unnecessary to chill the blocks. To insure rapid alloy setup, however, it would be advisable to use a water ring.

Chapter 6.
Generating

After blocking, allow the plastic lenses to sit one-half hour. This allows the lens, block, and alloy to stabilize to the same temperature. When everything is at the same (room) temperature, fewer "unexplainable deblockings" will occur. It was once thought that this one-half hour gave the alloy a chance to harden completely. However, if the proper base curve block is selected and chilled well, the alloy will be hardened throughout in far less than one-half hour. The problem is that the block is very cool, the alloy is very warm, and the lens is room temperature. The three should be given time to stabilize in temperature to avoid abnormal stress when they are pushed through the generator.

Variables—Plastic Lens

Ideally, plastic lenses should be generated with a special plastic diamond. This plated generator ring will allow you to remove much more material per pass, with less lens stress, than with the standard glass ring. It is not possible to use a plastic generator ring to cut glass lenses. Therefore, if you must cut both glass and plastic lenses on the same generator you will have to use a glass diamond. There are many glass generator rings on the market that attempt to compromise the two totally different cutting requirements, boasting to be all-around diamonds. If you have never had the opportunity to use an all-plastic setup to generate plastic lenses, you may even be impressed with the efficiency of the all-around diamond ring.

The speed and accuracy of generating can be greatly affected by the style of blocks and the computer system used. Some labs use the small standard Coburn glass blocks and remove 8 to 10mm per generator pass. The argument persists that when removing that much material with so small a block backing, the lens will bend, distorting the surface. However, those who are successfully using this system maintain that with an aggressive diamond and a top-running generator, the lens cuts freely and does not distort. They further maintain that those labs that make multiple generator passes per lens are inviting problems caused by heat buildup.

You can see there is a substantial amount of controversy as to which is the best system to use. There are some simple guidelines to follow when selecting the system that will best suit you. Remember that plastic lenses have raised segs on most of the multifocals. If you allow the seg to interfere with either the block or the generator ring, you will be inviting prism. When using the Coburn glass blocks you would be well advised to use an Ultex generator ring to go around the seg, regardless of its style. This is a very simple and accurate method to eliminate whatever prism-producing effect the seg could have.

Any prism that must be ground on the lens cannot be put on with a ring, but rather must be shimmed on with prism wedges. Although this system will work, a good deal of care must be exercised. As the prism wedges get thicker, the possibility for cross prism increases and productivity decreases. Therefore, using the small Coburn glass blocks with a computer system that uses on-center blocking will cause unnecessary problems at the generator. Add to this "system" a glass diamond in your generator, and you have probably the worst possible setup. The easiest way to clean up this mess would be to switch to a larger block or alloy backing system. This would encompass the seg, give a level surface for the prism rings, and a large backing to help eliminate lens bending.

There is no one correct method, but rather many systems that can be tailored to fit your needs. The important thing to remember is that every phase of your system affects the other phases. Compatibility is the key to productivity.

Whether to use oil or water-based generator coolant is an interesting question. Plastic diamond life is not affected as adversely as glass diamond life when using a water-based coolant rather than oil. With the cost of oil rising at an alarming rate, water-based coolant is also financially appealing. Unfortunately, there are some drawbacks to water-based coolants. The spray from generating constantly bathes your generator or at least its ways. While oil lubricates and fights rust, water does quite the opposite. If adequate maintenance is not performed, water-based coolant can turn your generator into a large piece of useless rust. Oil is still cheaper than a generator. Oil also has less tendency to foam. A centra cool and centrifuge will greatly enhance the efficiency of either method.

Chucking and Beveling Plastic

Chucking the lens may be the most important part of generating. Place the correct ring on the block. If you require prism, remember to align the arrowhead on the lens with the prism ring mark. Without allowing the prism ring to turn, place the lens in the generator chuck. Make sure the chuck is open all the way and is clear of any foreign substance. In most generator chucks you will find a pin at the top that fits into the block to retain axis. Slide the pin as far into the block as possible.

The block must be pushed toward the chuck with equal pressure all the way around it to avoid tipping the lens slightly and creating prism. This can be accomplished with substantial pressure using fingertips only on the lens that lies over the center of the block. If you use on-center blocking this is the center of the lens. To avoid tipping the lens, do not allow any other part of your hand to come in contact with the lens.

When everything is set the way you want it, close the chuck tightly around the block. You are now ready to generate. The steps in generating are based on the style of generator and will therefore be left to the manufacturer's operations manual.

When you have completed generating the lens, remove it from the chuck and immerse and clean it in a soap solution. This will remove the oil or generator coolant from the block and lens that would otherwise contaminate the finer.

Before proceeding to the finer, the lens should be beveled. The bevel serves two purposes: (1) the beveled lens is more apt to ride over the fining pads without tearing them, and (2) the bevel eliminates the sharp edges that could break off, possibly scratching or waving the lens surface. If at any time during the fining or polishing operations the bevel wears off, it should be redone.

Generating Glass

The basic principles behind generating plastic lenses also apply to glass lenses. After blocking, the temperature should be allowed to stabilize prior to generating. Once the lens, block, and alloy have stabilized to the same temperature (not necessarily room temperature), generating may proceed. This should not take more than five to ten minutes.

Variables

The type of diamond used will greatly affect generator performance. Diamonds are divided into several categories based on expected performance. The first category is a division based on coolant type. The use of oil or water-based coolant will affect the performance and life of the diamond.

The second category is concerned with the lens material being cut. Glass diamonds may be bought for cutting nonphoto, photo, or photo and plastic lenses. Each lens material creates special cutting needs.

The third category is diamond bond. In simple terms, the bond type is the metal used in conjunction with the diamond. It basically holds the diamonds to the surface of the generator ring. The speed at which a generator ring will wear out can generally be traced to the type of bond used. While a softer bond will tend to wear sooner, it will allow you to remove more material per pass.

The fourth category is slots, the cuts put into the diamond surface. The width and angle of these slots vary, depending on the manufacturer and your needs. They aid cutting and ring cooling.

The fifth category is diamond grit. This is simply the size of the diamond. Each manufacturer has its own designs, but basically these are the five factors that must be taken into consideration to produce the right diamond ring for you.

The most important aspect in generating glass is the coolant type and flow. Previously it was stated that a glass ring will wear faster using a water-based coolant. The rust problems inherent with water-based coolants were also noted. This sounds like a very convincing argument for oil coolant. However, there is one thing that oil can give you that water cannot when cutting glass—fire. Generating is the only place in the surface shop operation where heat creates more of a problem with glass than plastic lenses. Glass, a harder surface than plastic, creates more heat when generated. Photo glass is even hotter. The grinding chamber can get hot enough to ignite the oil. Most of the time these are little flashes, but large fires have destroyed an entire lab.

Now you are probably wondering why anyone would use oil. It goes back to the wear on the diamonds and the possibility of changing a generator into a rust pile with water-based coolant. If proper procedures are followed, there is no reason for the oil to ignite. The first precaution concerns the oil flow. The manifold spouts must direct the oil flow according to the diamond manufacturer's specifications. This can vary depending on the wheel slots and other design variables. Basically, most manifolds have three spouts, shown in Figure 10. One spout directs oil into the diamond hub for cooling. The other two spouts direct oil to the cutting surface at approximately the nine and eleven o'clock positions.

With the manifold spouts in place, your only other concern lies in the amount of oil flowing. Turn the flow on as fast as possible. How much is too much? If the generator's oil return overflows or backs up, turn the flow down until the return can just handle the flow. If you must wear waders to generate, the flow is probably a little much. Another thing to watch for is the cleanliness of your oil. Dirty oil is not nearly as effective a cutting or cooling agent as clean oil. Obviously the best cleanliness and cooling aid is the use of a centra cool and centrifuge. If an adequate flow of properly directed, clean, cool oil is used, you should be able to remove 5mm of photo glass per pass once the curve is set in the lens.

Chapter 7.
Fining and Calipering

It would be difficult to single out the one most important phase in the total lens fabrication system. Fining may not be the most important, but it is the phase that can make the most changes in the ultimate appearance of the finished lens. If the lens coming off the generator is too thick, has the wrong curve, or has a misplaced optical center, the finer can rectify the problem. The quality of the fine also determines to a great degree the success the polisher will have.

The more changes that can be effected by any phase of an operation, the more that can go wrong during that operation. With this in mind we should carefully examine each step of this operation.

Fining Systems

With plastic lenses, most people use cold tap water for their slurry. A fine of nominal grit can be used, but as you will see this can be unnecessarily expensive, messy, and hard on the machines.

The best type of pad to use is not nearly as clear-cut. The basic idea is a two-pad system. A first fine pad removes the generator marks and makes minor curve adjustments. This pad is 1,200-grit silicon carbide and is gray in color. After the lens has run on the first fine pad for from twenty seconds to one minute (depending on the quality of curve off of the generator and style and mechanical soundness of the cylinder machine), you are ready for the second fine pad (see Figure 11).

The second fine pad is 10 micron aluminum oxide and is yellow in color. Do not remove the first fine pad from the lap. Simply place the second fine pad exactly on the first fine pad. The cut of the pad should be the same, allowing the second fine pad to completely cover the first fine pad. The lens is usually run on the second fine pad for from 1½ to 2½ minutes, depending on the quality of surface left from the first fine pad and the cylinder machine. After the second fine is complete, remove both the first and second fine pads from the lap. Clean the lap carefully to remove any residual pad adhesive, and proceed to the polisher.

This is probably the most-used system, but it is far from the only system available. There are at least four different first fine grits and six different second fine grits available. Anything rougher than 1,200-grit first fine is generally black in color. The extremely rough first fine pads have the texture of a gravel pit.

These pads are used to extend the range of your generator, but they should be used carefully. Their aggressiveness can create thin lenses quickly, and their grit will contaminate the slurry. You need not even use that rough a pad to contaminate the slurry.

Many people use a black 600 grit for their first fine. This rougher pad is more forgiving of generator operator errors. You would be foolish not to have some 600 grit and even rougher pads in stock for emergencies, but to use them as your staple points to problems. Clean, cold water fines faster than warm, contaminated water. The water gets contaminated fast enough with plastic and fine 1,200 grit without making matters worse with 600 grit.

The second fine pad may not remove all of the scratches caused by loose, rough particles floating in the slurry. If these particles are pumped up near the end of the cycle, the second fine pad does not stand a chance. On occasion it will be necessary to use a rough pad. This, along with the natural buildup of contaminants, makes it necessary at times to change the slurry. These are the times that you will be glad you are throwing away inexpensive tap water rather than fine. The use of tap water allows you to change the water often enough to keep it cold—unless, of course, you have the worthwhile luxury of a slurry cooling system. Water is also easier on pumps, block centers, points, and in cleanup.

One-step pads in most cases do not work as well as the two-pad system. The one-step system must either give up the aggressiveness of the first fine pad or the smoothness of the second fine pad. The one-step pad that leaves an adequate surface for polishing generally will not make any curve change, will have difficulty with moderate to deep generator marks, and will take too long. The one-step pad that does a decent first fine will either leave too rough a surface to obtain a decent polish, thus extending the polish time, or take too long to fine, relying on the pad wear to change the grit from first to second fine. Some people have found this one-step system workable, and it bears experimentation on your part.

There are many other systems available. The friction grip system eliminates adhesive in favor of friction using a unique, semipermanent base pad. The diamond pad system replaces the first fine pad with a diamond-impregnated, semipermanent pad boasting up to 1,000 surfaces per pad. Another system features precut laps with a diamond-impregnated surface. These are but a few of the possibilities. Fortunately, most pad suppliers are happy to give you samples to help you determine what might be the best system for you.

Fining Machines, Tools, and Materials

Most people run spheres and cylinders on cylinder machines. The use of sphere machines in the plastic shop has become antiquated. The only argument remaining is whether or not you need to spin the sphere or not. For those who feel it is necessary to spin spheres, there are two ways to do it.

The first way is to use a sphere adapter. Using a special pin holder and block cap, the same machine used for cylinders can be used for spheres. Some people feel this adversely changes the pin-to-block angle, and they use the second method. This is simply to change the cylinder machine over to a one-pin sphere machine.

The theory behind spinning spheres is that this is the only way to insure not inducing cylinder. Depending on your equipment, this may not be true. If you have a good sphere tool cutter—one that spins the tool while cutting—it is difficult or impossible to create any cylinder in the tool. This good tool coupled with a well-maintained cylinder machine should not give you cylinder in your spheres, even if you do not spin them.

Aluminum versus Plastic Tools

The material the tools are made of is an important factor in the plastic shop. Cast iron tools, while good in the glass shop, have no business in the plastic shop. They are unnecessarily heavy, causing excessive wear on the cylinder machines; worst of all, they rust. Rust is one thing you do not need contaminating the fine and, especially, the polish. Aluminum and plastic are the alternatives. The choice between the two of them is difficult. The first plastic tools on the market did not hold curve well, although this problem seems to have been rectified.

Plastic tools will increase the life of your tool cutter and its tip because they are much easier to cut than either cast iron or aluminum. Care must be used when clamping a plastic tool down to be cut. If too much clamping pressure is used, the tool will bend. If the tool is checked immediately after it is cut, the curve may appear to be correct; several minutes later, however, after the tool has returned to shape, the curve will be flat. It does not take long to learn that since a plastic tool cuts easily, only moderate clamping pressure is needed; then your tool curves will look good.

Herein lies the strongest argument against using plastic tools. Through constant clamping on the cylinder machine lap tables, can we expect this possible bending to be enough to affect the lens' curve? The answer to that obviously has a good deal to do with how heavy the lap table clamping pressure is. Even if this were the case, the tools could be cut slightly flat to compensate for the bend if it were your desire to use plastic tools.

There is another good reason for using plastic tools: The pads can be removed much more easily from a plastic tool than an aluminum tool, and less adhesive remains on the tool. Plastic tools will therefore speed up both the pad removal and cleanup operations.

If you use a pad press, you have all the more reason to use plastic tools. It is very important to have the pads placed on the tools in a wrinkle-free manner. Even the smallest wrinkle can cause a wave in the lens. The steeper the tool curve, the more difficult it is to apply a wrinkle-free pad to the tool. If you use a pad press to apply the first fine pads, your problems will generally be over. It is seldom necessary to use the pad press to apply the second fine pad, although with some extremely steep curves this may be a good idea. It seems as though with every solution to a problem, a new problem arises. A pad press, while eliminating pad wrinkles, makes pads extremely difficult to remove. The solution is to use plastic tools. With plastic tools the pads are removed easily, but there could be curve problems. On and on it goes. That is why we must stress using a system, not individual phases. It simply cannot be said often enough: Each phase affects the others.

Glass Fining Powders

The fact that glass is a harder surface than plastic means that the surface will not fine as easily. Instead of using pure water, a grit slurry is necessary. Most labs currently use a form of aluminum oxide powder. When mixing the powder with water to form your slurry, attention should be paid to the manufacturer's Baumé and pH factor recommendations. These readings can vary substantially from product to product.

The discussion of glass fining powders closely parallels that of plastic fining pads. In both cases, various grits are made for the same reasons. Also in both cases, samples are available for your testing. Remember that a rough grit will curve the lens in more quickly but will also present a more difficult polishing task. In the case of spheres that are fined on a hand pan, multiple grits are generally used. You start with a rough grit to curve the lens in quickly and switch to a fine grit to speed polishing. This multiple grit idea is unnecessary with cylinders or spheres run on high-speed cylinder machines. Most labs are slowly switching to the plastic shop idea of running the glass spheres on cylinder machines.

Tools and Machines for Glass

Until now you saw a strong resemblance between the fining of glass and plastic lenses. The largest discrepancy lies in tools. Cast iron is by far the most-used tool material, because the lens is fined directly on the surface of the tool. Most other materials would wear too quickly due to the hardness of the glass and the grit of the slurry.

It is also possible to use metal fining pads on top of the tools. This way the pad wears, not the tool. Do not confuse metal glass-fining pads with the paper or plastic pads used to fine plastic. The glass pads are much harder to get on and remove. Some people argue that when pads are used, any kind of tool material will work.

There are several reasons why most labs do not use fining pads. Obviously, the first reason is the cost of fining pads. Along with the cost of the pad itself is the cost in downtime to change worn pads. Another reason not superficially obvious is in the polishing process cleanup. The adhesive on polish pads can leave a residue that requires removal by solvent. When the solvent is rubbed across the fining pad to remove the polish pad adhesive, the solvent may loosen the fining pad adhesive. This will obviously loosen the fining pad, shortening its life and creating more downtime for pad changes. The last reason most labs do not use fining pads again has to do with polishing. The tool should be carefully rinsed between the fining and polishing phases. The contamination of the polish with fine grit could be costly, as it is with plastic lenses. A fining pad is more difficult to clean, so it is far more likely that polish contamination will occur when fining pads are used. This is not to imply that fining pads should not be used. When the proper care is exercised, either system is satisfactory.

Whether you are working with glass or plastic, when a pad is used the curve must be compensated. Another compensation you may want to work into the glass tools is the index of refraction difference. All of this is covered in the section on tool compensations. Some labs that fine directly on the tool surface add a wear factor to the tool. The tool curve is increased up to 0.06, and they use that tool until it is weak up to 0.06. The tools are trued less, more material must be removed per trueing, and the lens powers are less stable. This is a standard that each lab must take upon itself to set.

Regardless of how the curve is cut, a bare tool needs to be scored. Scoring is simply lines cut into the face of the tool by machine or file to aid in the flow of slurry between the lens and tool. Score lines are generally put either diagonally across the tool or perpendicular to the base of the tool, as shown in Figure 12. Diagonal lines will move the slurry better, but they wear the tool more quickly. With the pumps available in today's finers, enough slurry flow can be obtained without resorting to diagonal scoring.

Glass fining is a one-step operation of approximately four to six minutes on the average high-speed cylinder machine. The time will vary depending on the machine, slurry, curve being fined in, and quality of curve off the generator.

Glass is less forgiving of generator-to-cylinder-machine curve differences than plastic. A plastic lens is more likely to bend and slowly fine in an off curve, while the brittle nature of glass is more likely to cause a breakage due to curve differences.

A lens that is coming in rough will make a distinctive sound. When you hear the additional noise you would be wise to stop the cylinder machine and check the lens. The lens should be checked two ways. First, make sure you have the correct lens on the correct tool. If so, examine how the curve is coming in. If the curve difference appears to be minor, switch the cylinder machine to a slower speed, and switch back to fast speed once the curve is in. If the curve difference is major, the lens should be regenerated to the correct curve (see Figure 13).

When regenerating, the same type of procedure used in removing prism can be used. That is, mark the surface of the lens with a red grease pencil, and, taking as little off as possible, slowly generate until the grease pencil is gone.

When the cylinder machine cycle is completed, inspect the lens. The lens should be free of all generator marks and have a smooth, clean surface. If this is not the case, the lens should be fined longer. If the lens passes the test, you may proceed to the polisher. Make sure that both the lens and tool have been rinsed thoroughly to remove the slurry.

Calipering

Prior to and during the fining of both glass and plastic lenses, calipering may be necessary. The only way calipering can be accurate is by making certain that the calipering points are equal distance from the center of the block. The easiest way to do this is by calipering directly on the lens, but up against the side of the block.

Specifically, through which meridians the calipering should take place depends on the lens curve. The types of curves and calipering points are summarized in Figure 14.

The first and simplest curve is a sphere without prism. A sphere should be exactly the same thickness at all points equidistant from the center of the block.

The second curve is a cylinder without prism. Think of a cylinder as two spheres crossed at right angles. You caliper this lens as though it were two spheres. The lens should be the same thickness equidistant from the center of the block through the meridian of least curve (base). Secondly, the lens should be the same thickness equidistant from the center of the block through the meridian of the most curve (cross). The thickness running through the base curve meridian will not be the same as the thickness running through the cross curve meridian.

The third type of curve is either spherical or cylindrical, with prism ground on it. You must first determine whether or not you have the correct amount of prism ground on the lens. You marked the prism meridian with an arrowhead line. Through this meridian the thickness difference must match the expected rise in prism thickness difference. This can be determined using the following formula:

$$d = \frac{L\Delta}{\mu - 1}$$

The difference in thickness is equal to the length of the prism in meters times the amount of prism divided by the index of refraction minus one. (The length of the prism is the distance between calipering points.)

For example, if the shop slip requires 4Δ on a glass lens of index 1.523, what should the thickness difference be if the calipering points are 48mm apart?

$$d = \frac{L\Delta}{\mu - 1}$$

$$d = \frac{(0.48)4}{1.523 - 1}$$

$$d = 3.671$$

Therefore, when calipering a glass lens of index 1.523 at 48mm, a 4Δ should measure 3.67mm thicker at the base than at the apex.

Although the formula is not very difficult, it would certainly be substantially easier if you could come up with a single number that when multiplied by the amount of prism would obtain the thickness difference. You can. Two of the variables in the formula can be eliminated for most computations. Especially in the glass shop, most people use only one diameter of block. And generally the index of glass used is 1.523. If the distance between the calipering points is 48mm, the magic number would be

$$\frac{0.48}{1.523 - 1} = 0.91778, \text{ or approximately } 0.92$$

Now all you need to do to obtain the approximate thickness difference is multiply the amount of prism times 0.92. For example,

$$4 \times 0.92 = 3.68$$

For blocks of different sizes or indexes, you will need to calculate a new magic number. A chart can be easily constructed using your magic number for your future reference.

After you have calipered through the prism meridian, you must caliper 90 degrees opposite that meridian. The thickness running through the meridian 90 degrees opposite the prism meridian should be the same equidistant from the center of the block.

This type of calipering will only work if the outside curves are the same at the points of calipering. Be careful where you caliper when working with executive, progressive, plastic, or other multifocals that have more than one outside curve.

Summary of Procedures

Whether you are fining glass or plastic, here are some basic steps to follow.

1. The lens should be rinsed thoroughly of all oil or water-based generator coolant.
2. A good bevel should be put on the lens to avoid chipping the lens and ripping the pad in the case of plastic lenses.
3. Carefully select the correct tool. In plastic, place a wrinkle-free first fine pad on the tool. In glass, if metal fining pads are used, inspect them for wear and change them if necessary. If a bare tool is used, check the curve and retrue and score if necessary.
4. Make sure the tool seats completely on the cylinder machine tool holder.
5. If necessary, caliper the lens to determine if unwanted prism exists. If so, offset accordingly.
6. The cylinder machine pins should put the pressure down in the geometric center of the lens. If the regular block centers do not lie in the geometric center of the lens, use the offset holes in the block or an offset adapter.
7. If a grit slurry is used, make sure its Baumé and pH are correct. If water is used, make sure it is as cool and uncontaminated as possible.
8. After selecting the correct operating time and speed, start the cycle.
9. If any unusual sounds occur, stop the machine, inspect, and correct.
10. If necessary, periodically stop the machine to caliper the prism removal progress and adjust.
11. When the cycle is finished, inspect the lens. In plastic, if the first fine passes, place the second fine pad on and cycle for its time. If a second fine passes, remove both pads, clean the tool, and proceed to the polisher. In glass, if the lens passes, clean the tool and proceed to the polisher.

Chapter 8.
Polishing

The polishing of plastic lenses presents fewer variables than fining; most systems fall in line at this point. This is a one-pad, one-cycle operation. The pad is soft, with a feltlike nap. The thickness and composition of the nap will vary depending on the manufacturer. The pad in the most commonly used fine-polish system is blue.

Polish comes in basically two forms—powder and liquid. The powder must be mixed with water and sometimes other liquids, while most liquid polish comes ready to use after a thorough shaking. There is no great advantage to either: The powder may save some initial expense, but you still have to pay someone to mix it.

Procedures

The polishing procedure is relatively easy. After cleaning the tool of adhesive and contaminants, carefully place the polish pad on the tool. The polish pad's consistency is not prone to creating wrinkles and therefore seldom needs pad press application. It is a good idea to wet the pad prior to placing the lens on it. The lens will be done after three to six minutes, depending on curve, surface preparation, and cylinder machine.

If the system is running correctly, an inspection is almost unnecessary. Do it anyway. As shown in Figure 15, check for surface aberrations—waves, unpolished areas, gray areas, and scratches. The lens may be repolished on the same pad for a short time if necessary. Changing polishing pads may be in order, but generally, if the problem is that bad, the lens should be returned to the finer for a quick first fine and normal second fine.

Increasing Polish Effectiveness

There are two things that can be done to extend the life and increase the effectiveness of the polish. First, keep the polish cool with a chiller. Second, filter the polish. While it would be nice to have the luxury of a chiller and filter, if you do not, even running the polish through fine mesh or cheesecloth would be a great help. This will trap small pieces of plastic and precoat that might otherwise be pumped up to the lens surface, possibly scratching it.

Some people feel that a Baumé reading is also a must. This simple test requires little time and effort. The gauge itself (Figure 16) is composed of two pieces: a narrow cylinder and a glass, thermometerlike gauge. Fill the cylinder with the polish and insert the gauge. The gauge will go into the polish only to a point. Where the polish meets the gauge, take the Baumé reading, a measurement of specific gravity. Perhaps an easier but less accurate explanation would be that we are measuring the thickness or density of the polish. As the polish is used, it will break down and register a lower Baumé. When the Baumé reading varies from the manufacturer's specifications, more polish should be added or the polish changed entirely. Keeping the polish up to the manufacturer's specifications can be an expensive operation. Most labs prefer to keep the polish filtered and cool, adding polish only as the level dictates and changing the polish only when contaminated. Even with this simple operation, widely diverging opinions exist.

Variables with Glass Lenses

The procedure for polishing glass lenses is very similar to the plastic procedure. Rather than repeating the procedure, let us concentrate on the few differences. Most glass polish pads have a much harder surface. It is a thin, stiff, paperlike surface in comparison to the thicker, more feltlike nap surface of the plastic polish pad. The exception to this is the thick felt-style pad used by some to polish glass spheres when separate sphere and cylinder systems are used.

The polishing time is a little longer with glass. Approximately six to eight minutes can be expected, based on the same factors that affect plastic lenses. Another difference lies in the polish consistency. While filtering and chilling seem to be less important with glass, careful monitoring of the Baumé level seems to be more important.

These are the basic differences. Most of the other differences are caused by the specific machine, polish, pad, or system used.

Any problems that may arise when polishing either glass or plastic can probably be rectified by considering some of the steps outlined at the end of the chapter on fining and calipering. More specifically, consider the steps that apply to the cleanliness of the lens and tool, the bevel, selection of the tool, placement of the tool and lens on the cylinder machine, and the condition of the slurry.

Chapter 9.
Deblocking and Cleaning

Deblocking generally can be accomplished by rapping the lens on a hard surface. If the lens seems to be adhering too well or it has a very thin edge, do not deblock it in this fashion. After all of that work, this is no time to take chances.

Solving Deblocking Problems

Simply place the lens in the reclaim tank until the alloy warms enough to let go. The 3M-Armorlite Surface Saver tape will easily peel off after the block is removed. Precoats can be just as cooperative. If the lens is deblocked shortly after it comes off the polisher, most precoats will peel off in one easy piece. If the lens is not deblocked immediately, the precoat will dry out, creating a more substantial cleanup problem. Acetone will generally remove most precoats, but at the expense of contaminating the acetone more rapidly than necessary, even when the lens is only quickly dipped.

Care of Blocks

After the lenses are deblocked, put the blocks in the reclaim tank. Do not run the reclaim tank any warmer than necessary. You will want the temperature in line so you may feel free to deblock lenses in it. Make very certain that all of the alloy is removed from the block, especially in the area of the edge. This is where residual alloy could cause prism on the next lens it blocks. Have a brush handy to quickly go around the block as it is removed from the tank if necessary.

Blocks can rust even when rust inhibitor is put into the reclaim tank water. Even most aluminum blocks have steel centers quite capable of rusting.

Therefore, dry them off with a towel or air gun after they cool down. Taking good care of your blocks requires little time, but it will pay off in the long run.

The reclaim tank should be drained and cleaned regularly. Cleaning, along with use of a rust inhibitor, will insure a long, trouble-free life for your tank.

Cleaning Precautions

Glass lenses will generally clean up if you rub them with your fingers under warm water. Any stubborn spots can be cleaned with acetone. Avoid the use of other glass cleaners, as many have ingredients that could leave a film on the lens. This film is valuable in fighting fog or static in a finished pair of glasses. However, it may affect the bond strength of the finish shop block. This could create off-axis lenses due to block slippage in the edger.

The lens may be dried with either an air dryer or soft cloth. Do not allow spots of water to evaporate on the lens, as the heat from the lens working with the minerals in the water can leave a mark on the lens that will not wipe off. These marks can generally be removed by polishing, but why create another step?

Plastic lenses could be cleaned the same as glass lenses. The only problem is that the excessive rubbing needed to clean the lens may scratch the surface. The use of acetone rather than water will limit the need for rubbing the surface. Submerge the lens in a pan of acetone, cleaning the surfaces gently with an acetone-soaked cotton ball. Dry the lens with a soft cloth. (Good-quality diapers work very well.)

Air dryers may also be used. The important thing to remember when using an air dryer on plastic lenses is to make certain that the air line is filtered and regulated. Most air lines have at least some water in them, even when a water trap is used. This water can cause rust in the system. If you use a filter on the air dryer and keep the air velocity to a minimum, the chances of foreign objects hurting the lens surface are slim. Put a filter on the dryer even if you have a filter on the compressor. The filter on the compressor should take care of most of the problems coming from the air tank. The filter on the dryer will take care of the air line from the compressor to the dryer and anything that might back up from another machine on the same air line.

Once your glass or plastic lens is clean, it is time to inspect it. Inspect the lens carefully, looking for gray areas, scratches, pits, and waves. Be very sure to remove everything from the surface of the lens. This is especially true with plastic lenses, where baking the lenses in an oven is becoming a standard practice. Precoat or other cleanable marks left on the lens prior to baking could be baked into the lens permanently.

In baking plastic lenses, the heat will remove any block marks and similar imperfections. The amount of time and temperature varies, depending on the hardness of the lens and other minor factors. Start with 200° F for ten minutes and adjust as needed from there. If you are having problems removing block marks, there are several places to check. Check the quality and mix of your precoat. Check the coolness of the blocks and the temperature of the blocker. If everything seems to check out adequately, you would be well advised to experiment with another manufacturer's lenses.

SECTION II

Miscellaneous
Surface Shop Procedures

Chapter 10.
Tool Compensation

When a pad is added to a tool, the radius of curvature is made larger and thus the curve changes (Figure 17). By calculating how much the radius of curvature has changed, the tool radius can be compensated so that the combination of tool and pad will yield the desired curve.

Radius of Curvature

To calculate the amount of radius change, you must first convert the diopter tool curve to radius of curvature. To that answer add the pad thickness to obtain the radius of curvature of the padded tool. Convert the total radius of curvature back to diopters to determine the diopter curve of the padded tool. The difference between the diopter curve of the padded and unpadded tool is the amount of compensation needed in the tool.

For example, calculate the tool curve compensation necessary for a 500/800 tool curve using plastic lens pads:

$$\text{Radius of curvature} = \frac{\mu - 1}{\text{diopter}}$$

The radius of curvature is equal to the index of refraction minus one, divided by the diopter value.

All tools are based on a 1.530 index. The formula simplifies to the following:

$$R = \frac{0.53}{D}$$

$$R = \frac{0.530}{5}$$

$$R = 0.106\text{m, or } 106\text{mm}$$

Add the pad thickness to the tool radius of curvature. In the example, we will use the standard 0.018-inch plastic pad thickness. The thickness must be expressed in millimeters. The conversion is inches times 25.4 equals millimeters: $0.018 \times 25.4 = 0.4572$.

$$
\begin{array}{r}
106.0000 \\
+ \quad 0.4572 \\
\hline
106.4572\text{mm, or } 0.1064572\text{m}
\end{array}
$$

By reapplying the formula, the diopter value will be obtained.

$$D = \frac{0.530}{R}$$

$$D = \frac{0.530}{0.1064572}$$

$$D = 4.978526581$$

This is the actual curve produced when you pad a 5.00D curve with a 0.018-inch-thick pad. The difference between this curve and the original curve is the amount the tool must be increased to obtain the desired 5.00D curve when padded with a 0.018-inch-thick pad.

$$\begin{array}{r} 5.0000 \\ -4.9785 \\ \hline 0.0215 \end{array}$$, or approximately 0.02

If the base curve of the tool is cut 5.02D, the padded result will be 5.00D.

Cylinder

Along with the 5.00D base curve, we need a 3.00D cylinder to obtain an 8.00D cross curve. With plastic tools, most labs put the cylinder plastic compensation in the tool rather than at layout. To compensate for plastic, simply multiply the amount of cylinder by 1.065. A 3.00D cylinder with plastic compensation becomes 3.195. The desired resultant cross curve is 5.00 + 3.195, or 8.195. Now you may proceed the same as before:

$$R = \frac{0.530}{8.195}$$

$$R = 0.064673581m, \text{ or } 64.673581mm$$

$$\begin{array}{r} 64.673581mm \\ + \; 0.4572mm \text{ pad thickness} \\ \hline 65.130781mm \end{array} \text{ total radius, or } 0.065130781m$$

$$D = \frac{0.530}{0.065130781}$$

$$D = 8.137473432$$

$$\begin{array}{r} 8.19500 \\ -8.13747 \\ \hline 0.05753 \end{array}$$, or approximately 0.057

If the cross curve of the tool is cut 8.195 + 0.057, or 8.252, the padded result will be 8.195D.

The tool should be marked as a 500/300. The curves cut on the 500/300 tool should be 502/825 when using compensation based on a 0.018-inch pad thickness. When grinding plastic lenses it has become a traditional to accept the rounded base curve obtained from the 1.065 plastic compensation at layout. This is the number used to cut the base curve on the tool. The cross curve can be cut exactly by putting the unrounded compensation in the tool rather than using the rounded cross curve figured at layout. The important thing is not to compensate twice.

Rule of Thumb

Plastic lenses have a tendency to come out weak. The exact reason as to why remains speculative. Most labs use some form of arbitrary compensation based on experience rather than optical or mathematical soundness. This is not to say I object to the compensation, but rather to point out its true origin. A rough rule of thumb would be to start by adding 0.01 to a 2.00D curve and increasing the compensation 0.01 per diopter; e.g., 2.00 + 0.01 = 2.01; 3.00 + 0.02 = 3.02; 4.00 + 0.03 = 4.03, and so forth. This compensation should be added to the base curve only. The pad thickness compensation should be based on the original curve prior to adding our "mystery" compensation.

Glass pad thickness compensation is done exactly like plastic pad thickness compensation. Simply plug in the appropriate pad thickness and run through the formulas in the same way.

Index of Refraction

There is one other compensation that many people neglect: the index of refraction compensation. With plastic it was necessary to compensate by 1.065 at layout or in the tool. This number was obtained as follows.

$$\frac{1.530 - 1}{1.498 - 1} = 1.065$$

Glass compensation can be obtained by the following calculations:

$$\frac{1.530 - 1}{1.523 - 1} = 1.01$$

This compensation (1.01) is far less than the plastic compensation (1.065), but it definitely affects the higher powers. If you grind a −12.00D curve on a plano base lens 2mm thick, you will not get a −12.00D-powered lens. You will get a −11.87D-powered lens. The curve needed to obtain a −12.00D would be −12 × 1.01, or −12.12. Both base and cross curves must be compensated in this manner. Again, compensate for this at layout or in the tool, but not both places. You will find that most computers automatically calculate this and all of the needed compensations for both glass and plastic.

Chapter 11.
Vertex Change

The distance a lens sits away from the eye is referred to as the *vertex distance.* If the vertex distance changes, the effective power of the lens in relation to that eye will also change. This is why it is necessary to adjust the distance a magnifying glass is from the eye to obtain the optimum focus. While the ability to alter effective power by changing vertex distance is useful with a magnifying glass, it can be detrimental to spectacles. If the lens's vertex distance in the instrument used to examine the eye differs from the lens's vertex distance in the finished spectacles, an effective power difference will result.

Calculating Effective Power of a Lens

A very simple formula can be used to calculate the effective power of a lens with any amount of vertex change:

$$E = \frac{P}{1 \pm VP}$$

The effective power is equal to the prescribed power divided by one plus or minus the vertex change in meters times the prescribed power.

You use the plus sign in the denominator of the formula if you are dealing with a plus lens moved away from the eye or a minus lens moved toward the eye:

$$E = \frac{P}{1 + VP}$$

You use the minus sign in the denominator of the formula if you are dealing with a plus lens moved toward the eye or a minus lens moved away from the eye:

$$E = \frac{P}{1 - VP}$$

As an example, what is the effective power of the prescription $-11.00 - 3.00 \times 90$ if the refractive distance were 13mm and the wearing distance 15mm? We will use the formula with the minus sign in the denominator, because what we have is a minus lens being moved away from the eye.

$$E = \frac{P}{1 - VP}$$

$$E = \frac{11}{1 - (0.002)(11)}$$

$$E = 11.2474$$

Therefore, the spherical part of the effective power prescription is -11.25.

To obtain the cylindrical part of the effective power prescription, do not apply the formula to -3.00. The cylinder amount in a prescription is not a power; it is rather a difference of power between the strongest and weakest meridians. In this case, one meridian is -11.00 and the other meridian is -14.00. The formula should be applied to the -14.00 to determine the effective power through the strongest meridian:

$$E = \frac{14}{1 - (0.002)(14)}$$

$$E = 14.4039$$

Therefore, the effective power through the strongest meridian is -14.37. The amount of cylinder is the difference between the weakest and strongest meridians, which in this case is the following:

$$
\begin{array}{r}
-14.37 \\
- \quad -11.25 \\
\hline
-\ 3.12
\end{array}
$$

Therefore, the effective power of the prescription $-11.00 -3.00 \times 90$ moved 2mm away from the eye is $-11.25 -3.12 \times 90$. The axis of the prescription is in no way affected by a vertex change.

Chapter 12.
Removing Prism

A lens is said to have unwanted prism if the optical center lies other than where you desire it. In order to remove this prism you must determine two things: its amount and direction.

How Much and Where?

The amount of prism Is measured using a Lensometer. Place the lens in the Lensometer where the OC should be, and read the amount of unwanted prism created. This diopter value must then be translated into millimeters of thickness error. This thickness error is accounted for by the rise in prism and can be easily measured with the lens calipers. You will be using the calipers on both sides of the block through the axis where the prism lies to determine if you have removed it. The chart will give you a thickness difference, according to the diameter of the block of which you are calipering either side of and the amount of prism to be removed. The diameter is based on where the calipering will take place. Remember to consider not only the diameter of the block, but also any other factor that may move the calipering points farther apart; for example, alloy around the block, as in the Coburn glass blocking system that runs a ring of alloy around the block.

Now that you know the amount of thickness to remove, you must find out from where it is to be removed. Do not concern yourself with the base of the prism created by the error. What you need to know is the direction the OC must go to neutralize the error. Say you need to move the OC up. Whether the lens is minus or plus will determine what you must do to move the OC (see Figure 18). To move the OC up on a minus lens, you would have to remove lens thickness from the top of the lens. However, to move the OC up on a plus lens, you would have to remove lens thickness from the bottom of the lens. The rule of thumb is "minus pulls and plus pushes." Remember that a lens is not necessarily plus or minus throughout the lens. A lens can be plus in one meridian and minus in another. Check your lens to see if it is plus or minus in the meridian where the prism is to be removed.

Blocking and Calipering

Now that you know how much thickness to remove from which side of the lens, you are ready to remove the prism. Along with the normal lens markings, put an asterisk (*) where the prism is to be removed. The selection of cold blocking or alloy blocking is based on the normal parameters. The location of a multifocal lens on the block will vary, depending on what is to be done to the lens. If the lens is to be generated, you must mark and block the lens as you did initially, using either the standard or on-center method. If the lens is to be fined and polished only, it should be blocked on center. Single-vision lenses will, of course, be blocked on center.

After blocking using the appropriate system, the lens should be calipered. You will need to find two calipering points, on the side near the asterisk and the other 180 degrees opposite. The block makes an ideal reference, since the calipering points must be equidistant from the center of the block. If the lens size allows, caliper next to and on both sides of the block. If this is not possible, move both points equally in or out from there. If you prefer, with wide-throat calipers it is possible to caliper directly on the block.

Caliper and write down the thicknesses of the two points. In most cases the side with the asterisk will be thicker, but this is not always the case. Also, do not expect the amount of material to be removed to always balance the thickness at the calipering points. The thickness to be removed is the amount the rise in prism is incorrect. This thickness, therefore, must be removed from the asterisk side only. This is why we caliper 180 degrees opposite the asterisk. For example, say the calipering points measure asterisk side, 4.3; 180 degrees opposite, 3.7. We need to remove 0.4 to relocate the OC correctly. On our first attempt we remove exactly 0.4, and the asterisk side reads 3.9. Checking the other side, we find 3.6. Although we removed 0.4 from the asterisk side, the difference only changed 0.3, because 0.1 was removed from the opposite side. We would have to continue trying until the difference changed 0.4.

Generating and Fining

There are two ways to remove prism: The prism may be either generated or fined off. It is easier to remove a large amount of prism on the generator than the finer. Prior to chucking the lens in the generator, draw multiple lines with a grease pencil on the lens. Set the generator to remove 0 to 0.1, and make a pass. Checking the grease pencil lines will indicate how the curve is changing. The curve change may also be felt by hand. Continue making small takeoff passes until you have the new curve across the lens. Do not take off any more material than necessary. Determine how large a lens is needed. It may not be necessary to put the new curve all the way across the lens. When you have completed generating the lens, it should be fined and polished normally.

Both large and small amounts of prism can be removed on the finer. Smaller amounts of prism are more readily removed using the finer than the generator. This prism may be removed by offsetting the lens, putting more pressure on the asterisk side using the offset holes in the block or an offset adaptor. If more pressure is needed, push with your thumb on the asterisk side while fining. All you are trying to do is make one side more aggressive than the other. Another way to make one side more aggressive is by using two different types of grit fining pads. Cut a rough and a fine grit pad in half so that when placed on the tool, they lie opposite the prism axis. Place the rough grit half pad on the tool under the asterisk side, and put the fine grit opposite it. This will rapidly change the difference between the two calipering points.

Couple the pad idea with an offset adaptor, and you will make major changes rapidly. Do not get too carried away, though, because the curve must be brought across the lens. After most of the difference has been fined out, you should switch to the one-pad system to bring the curve across. Once you have achieved a smooth curve, along with the correct thickness reduction, proceed normally to the second fine and polish.

Chapter 13.
Cold Blocking and Reruns

Variables in Reruns

After inspecting the lens, you may decide it must be rerun. Which blocking method should you use? With a plastic lens, heat is now the biggest concern, as it was when you initially blocked the lens blank. Then the heat was dissipated throughout the thickness of the lens. After the lens has been through the surface shop, however, it is much thinner. If the lens is too thin, the heat will concentrate rather than dissipate and will damage the lens probably beyond repair.

When is a lens too thin to block on alloy? The answer lies in how good an alloy blocking system you employ. The use of chilled blocks in conjunction with maintaining as cool an alloy temperature as possible will greatly extend the operating range of your alloy blocking system. With properly controlled temperatures, you can expect to alloy block all plastic lenses over 3mm center thickness—provided you use the smallest blocks possible. Obviously, the less alloy used, the less heat created and the better the results. Cold blocking is used when the lens is too thin or you would rather not take chances.

Cold Blocking Plastic Lenses

Cold blocking is, basically, gluing the lens to the block. The system is composed of four parts: two types of resins, spacer disks, and blocks. Prior to cold blocking, a lens should be precoated in a normal manner. After the precoat is dry, place spacer disks on the lens. There are three reasons for using the spacer disks to raise the lens off the surface of the block. First, the disks create the recommended resin depth. Second, when placed properly, the disks assure multifocal segment clearance as well as proper executive and other nonstandard lens blocking. (See Figure 19.) Improper placement of the spacer disks could create prism if the cold-blocked lens is generated. Third, the space created by the disks will greatly facilitate deblocking.

After placing the spacer disks on the lens, you are ready to mix the resin. Most people mix the resin directly on the block. Pour equal amounts of each resin into the middle of the proper base block. Stir the resins together. The more vigorous and complete the mixing, the more quickly the compound will harden. Incomplete mixing of the compounds will result in excessive hardening time. Push the mixed compound toward the middle of the block as you complete the stirring. Set the block on a flat surface and place the lens on it. Press the lens down until it bottoms out on the spacer disks. The compound mounded up in the center of the block will have moved out toward the edge of the lens in a uniform manner, without any voids.

At this time there is nothing further to do except to make sure that the lens is on axis and wait for the compound to harden. A proper blocking job will have compound under as much of the lens as possible without excessive overflow. Mixing the correct amount of compound initially is the trick.

If you have many cold blocks to do, you may want to set them all up at once. Precoat and apply the spacer disks to all of the lenses. Place all of the necessary blocks on a flat surface near the lenses. In a separate container, mix a large batch of compound. After the compound is thoroughly mixed, pour some into the center of each block, and then place the lenses on the blocks. There are only two disadvantages with this "production" system. Waste can occur more easily if you mix too much compound. Second, with many lenses the compound might harden on the block before you can place the lens on it. With experience and skill, however, either method should work satisfactorily.

When the compound has hardened, proceed in a normal fashion through the shop procedures until deblocking. If a thick enough lens hangs over the block, you may wish to knock it off normally. However, in most cases it is better to proceed in a different manner. Most labs pry the lens off. Simply place a dull dinner knife between the block and the compound, and pry. Notice that the prying is not done between the lens and a compound; this could scratch the lens. Even if you pried at several spots around the lens, you could break a thin lens.

A better removal method is heat. Place the blocked lens in the reclaim tank for a few minutes, and then pry. The lens will practically fall off. There is another advantage: The heat has turned the compound into a soft, rubbery mass. The compound can be easily removed in one piece from the block with the same dull knife. Keeping the blocks this clean will be quite an advantage for future blocking.

Alloy Blocking Glass and Plastic Lenses

Since glass lenses do not suffer from heat-related problems, alloy blocking should be used for all reruns on them. Most labs have permanently discarded the old pitch block method. Basically, pitch blocking is gluing the lens to a block using heat and pitch. Both the block and lens must be heated, generally with a torch. When they reach the proper temperature, pitch—melted in the flame of the torch—is dripped onto their surfaces like wax from a candle. Then the pitch is reheated on the block and the lens turned over onto the soft pitch. Pitch blocking has been discontinued because there are too many places for error, the process is too slow, and it requires too much training and technique compared to alloy blocking.

If you need to alloy block a small glass or plastic lens, it may be necessary to reduce the size of the alloy backing. If the lens is smaller than the block diameter, alloy will run out. To avoid this, some labs use clay or a finger to block the alloy flow. Another method is to place an O-ring inside the block but around the outside of the blocker spout. The lens and O-ring will form a seal and keep the alloy from leaking out.

Positioning

Regardless of the type of blocking system, one factor remains constant for either glass or plastic lenses. How a lens is positioned on the block is determined by what you intend to do to the lens. If it is necessary to regenerate, the lens must be blocked as it was initially. If the lens is going directly to the finer, it should be blocked on center. The axis line on the lens should be parallel to, but not necessarily over, the axis on the block. With on-center blocking it is easier to make the necessary rerun changes without the fear of inducing unwanted prism.

Give some thought to the blocking method, because how you block the lens can have a substantial effect on the success of your rerun.

Chapter 14.
High Minus

When the inside curve of a minus lens is excessively steep, consider alternative lens designs. The three most common alternatives are double concave, myodisc, and minus lenticular (Figure 20).

Double Concave

A double concave is a full-field lens with a minus curve on both sides. Some manufacturers make both semifinished single-vision and multifocal lenses with various minus fronts. There are several advantages to making your own single-vision minus fronts. You have added expense if you decide to stock minus fronts. If you order out all your minus fronts, you have added delay.

The very same thick, flat base lenses you normally stock for high minus is what you need to make minus fronts. Therefore, there is no added stock, expense, or delay. Making a minus front is no different than any other surface. Take off as little material as possible to obtain the necessary field size, and proceed normally.

The only trick to using a double concave for a prescription lies in the selection of front curve. This depends a great deal on your equipment and the needed field size. It is not necessary to use the least minus front possible; do not create fabricating problems. Within reason, steepen the minus on the front so that you are not using every piece of machinery in the shop to its capacity: How high will your generator cut? How steep a tool will the tool cutter cut? How difficult will it be to place wrinkle-free pads on the tool? By simply increasing the amount of minus on the front, you can make a difficult job easy.

The other problem is field size. As the curve steepens, the field size lessens. Increasing the minus front steepness flattens the inside curve, thus increasing the field size. Minus fronts generally start around −2.00 or −3.00D and run all the way up to splitting the total curve between the front and back. You can expect to get into the −20.00's, with up to a −12.00 curve on both sides of the lens. In a small enough eye size, this could give you a full-field lens. It will be extremely thick, however, since the curves are going away from plano at the same rapid rate. The only way this lens can be made thinner is to reduce the field size, making a myodisc.

Myodisc

A myodisc has a plano front or carrier with the high minus curve or bowl cut into the middle of the lens only. Most labs cut a bowl of approximately 38mm, although there is no reason not to vary the bowl size based on the size of the frame, the prescription, the doctor's request, or for fabrication ease. Work with the bowl side of the myodisc first. Since it is not going full field, you can put quite a bit of minus in the bowl. Try to take enough to allow the other side curve to be full field.

After the front side is done, finish the myodisc like the double concave, by running the needed inside curve. When you realize how much the thickness was reduced by going from the double concave's minus front to the myodisc's plano carrier, you will be tempted to reduce the thickness even more by going to a plus carrier. Some labs waste a great deal of time rolling and polishing the myodisc's plano carrier to a plus carrier. It would be a good deal simpler to use a minus lenticular.

Minus Lenticular

A minus lenticular is almost the same as a myodisc: The difference lies in the carrier curve. Instead of starting with a plano lens, start with a full-field cataract lens. As an example, grind the bowl in the middle of a 12 base hyper. All procedures are the same as with the myodisc, but what you achieve is the thinnest possible high minus lens. There actually is little or no reason for using the myodisc. If it is necessary to use a bowl rather than full field, you may as well use the thinnest possible lens—the minus lenticular.

The Bowl

The location, shape, and size of the bowl are all factors you can control. When we discuss location we are referring to whether the bowl will appear on the inside or outside of the finished glasses. Grinding the bowl on the inside with the full-field side of the lens facing outward makes a more aesthetically appealing pair of glasses, and this is the preferred location.

The bowl shape is a far more interesting factor. Most bowls are round, and the only way a bowl can be round is by using a spherical curve. Therefore, you must grind all of the cylinder on the full-field side of the lens. Although this is the most common method, consider what might happen if you incorporated the cylinder into the bowl: The bowl would appear oval instead of round. The longest dimension of the bowl would be through the weakest power's axis; that is, -18.00 -3.00 $\times$ 180. The -18.00 would run through the 180-degree meridian, while -21.00 would run through the 90-degree meridian.

In this case, if the cylinder were ground in the bowl, you would end up with an aesthetically appealing lens. If the frame's A measurement were larger than the B measurement, as is generally the case, it would be wise to incorporate the cylinder into the bowl if the weakest meridian is at 180 degrees. This will reduce the amount of carrier around the bowl, which will accomplish two things: (1) the bowl will become less obvious, and (2) the field of vision will increase. If you are going to grind the cylinder into the bowl, remember to consider how the angle of the bowl will look in the finished glasses. To avoid account rejection, you may want to use a spherical bowl with a larger diameter rather than an oval bowl.

That brings us to the last controllable factor—size. The larger the bowl size, the nearer you approach a double concave. Size increase is good in that it increases the field of vision. Unfortunately, an increase in bowl size has two bad effects: (1) The larger the bowl, the thinner the surfaced lens. You may not have enough thickness left to grind the curves on the other side of the lens. (2) The larger the bowl, the thicker the finished lens.

How do you know what the correct size should be? There are several factors to consider: the account's request, the frame size, how the lens will look in the frame, and the amount of power. There is no one correct size. A bowl may be any size; however, the normal range is 40 to 48mm. The most-used sizes are in the 42 to 44mm range. Carefully select the location, shape, and size of the bowl. It is in this selection that the quality of the finished glasses is determined.

Account Relations

The style of high minus lens you select will have a tremendous effect on the field size and thickness of the final product. No one lens is the best answer. Do not be afraid to call the account. Open lines of communication can be most helpful when dealing with the unusual prescription. It would be foolish for you to do the "impossible," making the prescription full field only to have the account return it. The account will simply use the hindsight advantage and point out that the lens is too thick and should "obviously" be done in minus lenticular form. This is the same account that will return the next prescription because it "obviously" should have been made full field regardless of thickness, rather than the minus lenticular you sent. "Account Relations" in the Appendix explores this problem.

Chapter 15.
High Plus

Plus lenses may be fabricated on either spheric or aspheric front lenses, as shown in Figure 21. Spheric front curve lenses are used in most non-postcataract applications. The curve on a spheric lens remains stable from the central zone to the periphery. Aspheric lenses have mostly postcataract applications. The curve on an aspheric lens flattens toward the periphery. The amount and rate of flattening varies among manufacturers. This flattening of the front curve greatly enhances peripheral vision by reducing the distortion inherent in high plus lenses. Flattening is referred to as drop, as in "3 drop" or "4 drop" lenses.

Spheric Front

Low- and mid- plus power lenses up to 8.00 to 10.00D can be satisfactorily fabricated on a spheric front. The 5.00 to 6.00D range is generally where peripheral distortion will first be noticed, especially in a very large lens. Other than for obvious reasons of thickness and weight, the possible peripheral distortion is another reason for dispensers to discourage very large eye sizes with this amount of correction. If an account complains of peripheral distortion in a mid- to high-plus-power lens, you should ask several questions. First, has the prescription changed much? The plus power may have increased through the meridian where the complaint lies. Second, has the eye size changed? Even a slightly larger eye size, especially coupled with a prescription change, can cause a large problem. Third, if there has been a frame change, how does the new frame sit on the patient with respect to the old glasses? A change in vertex distance, tilt, or face form would make a difference. Fourth, in the case of high plus, has the style of lenses changed from aspheric to spheric? Fifth with little or no change in prescription, was the base curve changed? This would substantially alter the inside curve, the last refracting surface before light hits the eye and thus the most influential surface with regard to image quality. Changes in the inside curve can be tolerated the least by most patients. Any one or a combination of these factors can make a difference in how the patient sees. The higher the plus, the greater the effect.

Fabrication

Low- and mid-plus-powered lenses fabricated on spheric fronts are run through the lab similarly to minus lenses. The basic difference is how the lens thickness affects the various operations. The thickness of a plus lens determines its diameter (Figure 22). Be careful when using a blocking system that employs various diameters of blocks or backings. The generated or fined lens could be substantially smaller than the lens blank you are starting with.

To avoid generating or fining a block, consider the eye size, strap thickness, and inside curve of the finished lens. The eye size and strap thickness will give you an idea of how thick the lens will be at what size. The flatter the inside curve, the more likely damage will occur at slightly beyond the eye size. Generator diamonds are too expensive to ruin because of a bad guess. If there is any question whether the correct block was selected, check the lens in the generator after only part of the thickness has been removed. The experience obtained by checking lenses will develop into a knowledge that does not require guessing.

Depending on the range of your generator, the lens may get smaller yet on the finer. If the final curve to be put on the lens is flatter than your generator will cut, you can expect all of the curve to come off the edges of the lens. This will reduce the diameter of the lens. To be properly fined and polished, lenses should have a substantial edge bevel. The thin, sharp edges of plus lenses make the bevel all the more important. In the case of the lens with a curve coming off the edge, the bevel will be fined away. Put the bevel back on the lens as often as it comes off. This will help prevent broken and scratched lenses.

In the redo operation, the thickness of the lens affects the necessary inside curve. If it becomes necessary to rerun a lens because of a wave, scratch, or some other reason, consider how much the lens thickness will be reduced, and adjust the inside curve. With experience you will be able to judge how long and on which fining pad a lens will need to be run to correct the problem. Pad suppliers can give you an accurate removal rate for their pads. Combining this information will give you the amount thickness will be reduced. In general, you will not be reducing the thickness enough to drop the tooling unless the original thickness was just enough to increase the initial tooling. Keep this inside curve thickness relationship in mind when a lens is found to be slightly off power. A thin or thick lens could be the reason for a power variance. For a thin lens, flatten the tooling; for a thick lens, just thin it out.

Aspheric Front

High plus lenses are generally fabricated on aspheric front lenses. Aspheric lenses are divided into two categories: full field and lenticular. (See Figure 21.) A full-field lens has correction over the entire diameter of the lens. It differs from regular lenses only in that it is aspheric rather than spheric. A full-field aspheric lens rapidly becomes thicker and heavier as the plus power increases. The only way to cut down the thickness and weight is by reducing the lens diameter. This can be accomplished by either limiting the eye size of the frame or the field size of the lens.

A lens composed of a limited field size surrounded by a carrier lens is called a lenticular. Its correction is limited to the field or bowl of the lens. The carrier of the lens only fills out the eye size; it has no optical value to the patient. There are two basic bowl designs: round and oval. The round bowl is generally 40mm in diameter, and the oval bowl measures 45mm horizontally and 40mm vertically. Since most frames have a larger A than B measurement, the oval bowl fills out the frame in a more aesthetically pleasing manner. Both bowl designs are available in single-vision, flat top, and round segment designs.

The layout of either full-field or lenticular aspheric lenses can be accomplished by computer or by hand. Each manufacturer has a recommended method to compute the inside curve and thickness for its lens. Although it is much slower than a layout computer, adequate results are obtained by carefully following their instructions.

The same problems and fabricating procedures associated with the low- and mid-plus range can be expected, in some cases on even a larger scale. The selection of a full-field or lenticular-style lens is based on many factors. However, if the account has made a selection that you feel will make an optically or aesthetically unsound pair of glasses, do not hesitate to inform them. Some manufacturers give parameters for the successful dispensing of their lenses. Accounts who insist on violating these parameters cannot expect a lens to function as it was designed. Most manufacturers have refracting, dispensing, and fabricating manuals that can be of use to you and your accounts.

Chapter 16.
Extending Your Generator Range

The popular 71, 75, and 80mm lens blanks forced labs to switch from 3- to 3½-inch generator diamonds. Unfortunately, this substantially reduced the operating range of the generator. One of the standard generators was the 390; with a 3½-inch diamond its range is 3.00 to 11.00D. Some labs are trading in their 390s for more sophisticated plano-to-20.00D range generators. If you need the added speed of most of these generators, their purchase could be a good idea. But to purchase one simply for its added range is foolhardy.

Adding Range—Pros and Cons

Extending the range from 3.00D down to plano can cause more harm than good. Most of these very flat curves are for very-high-plus-power lenses going into small frames. Cutting a very flat curve on a small lens should signal danger to you. The flatter the curve on a small lens, the more likely the generator diamond will be ruined cutting through a block, alloy, or generator ring. This ability to cut flat could cost you a great deal of money. Cutting the 3.00D curve and fining the lens in from there reduces this possibility. When you fine, the curve comes off the edge. This means there are no center thickness compensations to make, no calipering while fining, no problems at all. In the case of plastic lenses, which are more likely to be in this range, the selection of the correct fining pad will curve in the lens in no time at all. In short, buying a generator to cut flatter than 3.00D could be buying trouble.

On the other end of the scale the story changes completely. The ability to cut steeper curves can be very advantageous. When you cut flatter than the needed curve you must fine the curve in from the center out. This reduction in center thickness must be compensated for to avoid a thin lens. The amount of compensation depends on the needed field size and inside curve. Most people prefer to allow 1mm per diopter rather than spend the time to do the calculations. For example, say your generator cuts to 11.00D and you need to cut a 13.00D curve. The difference is 2.00D. You would remove 2mm less, leaving the lens 4mm thick instead of 2mm thick. Use an overall caliper to determine the thickness of the blocked lens in the center. Fine the lens, checking it periodically until you have removed 2mm. This is a workable but very slow process. The problem would have been solved if you could have used a 3-inch or smaller diamond.

Solutions—Expensive to Homemade

At least one manufacturer has come up with an expensive, semipractical solution to the problem. This system consists of a new Quickset and three special diamonds. The Quickset has three sets of numbers corresponding to the three different diamonds. This system has excellent range, but to maintain the system your "family" of diamonds must be kept to exact specifications. The standard 3½-inch glass diamond will wear or require retrueing far faster than the other two. This will change the relationship between the three wheels, forcing you to either guess at the curve, fine much longer, or needlessly retrue the whole family at once. It does not appear to be a financially sound system for glass. By comparison, the wear factor with plastic lenses is negligible. The relationship between the three diamonds will remain stable long enough to make the system very workable.

Several problems that in themselves do not negate the value of the system do bear examination. The three small sets of numbers on the Quickset could lead to operator error. If one of the diamonds is damaged or worn, you will have to obtain a replacement from the original company to maintain the diamond relationship. You lose the competitive market advantages of delivery time, quality control, and cost. Finally, the system is more expensive than is necessary.

A similar system for plastic can be set up for the cost of the diamonds only. If your 3½-inch diamond is good, simply purchase a 3-inch diamond. Now make a simple paper chart showing the corresponding 3-inch curve to the 3½-inch Quickset. For example, cut a sample lens at 11.00D with the 3-inch diamond. Measure the obtained curve with a lens clock or brass gauges. Put this result on the chart under the 3-inch diamond across from 11.00D. Now cut 10.50, then 10.00 and so forth, indicating your results on the chart. It will only take a few minutes and one lens (since you are cutting flatter each time) to develop a "system." If the 3-inch diamond does not cut high enough, purchase a smaller diamond and expand your chart. Simply hang the chart on the wall or tape it to the generator, and you are ready to go.

The advantages to this system correspond exactly to the disadvantages of the expensive system. Most of the work is done on the 3½-inch diamond. With only the 3½-inch numbers on the Quickset, operator error is reduced. A replacement diamond can be obtained from any source, so you retain your consumer advantages. It will simply cost you one lens and a few minutes to redo the chart. Finally, the cost is very reasonable.

This inexpensive system may also be used in glass by redoing the chart as wear or retrueing occurs. Depending on the number of times you find it necessary to switch diamonds to cut higher curves, there may be a simpler method. Instead of constantly redoing the chart, eliminate the chart altogether. When it becomes necessary to use the 3-inch diamond, use the sample lens. With a little experience it will only take a few cuts to obtain the desired curve. The sample lens and a few minutes is far better than fining and calipering half the day. Whether you are setting up a chart or using a sample lens, it is better to be a little steep than a little flat. This will only take a few seconds longer to fine, and it will all come off the edge.

Neither the expensive nor homemade system is perfect. Which one is best for you depends on your situation. In any case, you need not buy a new generator simply to expand your generator range. The expensive system is quite inexpensive by comparison. These systems are based on the 390 generator, but do not be afraid to experiment with any generator. You will probably find that it has a hidden range also.

Chapter 17.
Calculating an
Overrefraction

Some ophthalmologists and optometrists prefer to perform refractions while patients are wearing their glasses. This is generally referred to as over-refraction. The power obtained is not the final power, but rather the amount to be added to the patient's present prescription. For each eye there will be two prescriptions: the old prescription and the prescription to be added to it to obtain the total necessary power.

There are three ways to figure the final power. The first method is for those who wish to avoid working with numbers. Grind a lens with the power of the old lens and a lens with the difference power. Put the two lenses together in the Lensometer, and read the power. The accuracy of this system is obviously in question, but it may serve those who cannot work with numbers adequately. The second, graphic solution is the least recommended. It requires the use of basic geometry and algebra, and the reliability of its results are questionable. The third method is by formula. While it does require a bit more algebra, it does not require geometry and its results are considered by far the most accurate. Thompson's formula is one of the most reliable algebraic methods.

Thompson's Formula

There are three equations or steps used in Thompson's formula: one step each for calculating the sphere, cylinder, and axis of the resultant prescription. The equations follow, in order of use.

1. $C^2 = A^2 + B^2 + 2AB\cos2\Theta$
2. $\sin2\phi = \dfrac{B}{C}\sin2\Theta$
3. $S = \dfrac{A + B - C}{2}$

This is where:
C = the power of the resultant cylinder;
A = the power of the original or added cylinder (whichever has the smaller axis);
B = the power of the original or added cylinder (whichever has the larger axis);
Θ = the difference between the B and A axis (B axis − A axis);
ϕ = the angular amount to be added to the A axis to obtain the resultant axis; and
S = the amount the cylinders affect the final sphere power. (This answer must be added to the sphere powers of the original and added prescriptions to obtain the resultant sphere power.)

Both prescriptions should be in the same cylinder form. Either minus or plus cylinder will work.

An Example

It is much easier to understand this method if we consider an example:

$$Pl \; +4.00 \times 80 \quad \text{(original prescription)}$$
$$+1.00 \; +1.75 \times 135 \quad \text{(added prescription)}$$

A = +4.00   (the cylinder amount with the smaller axis)
B = +1.75   (the cylinder amount with the larger axis)
Θ = 55   (B axis − A axis)

1. $C^2 = A^2 + B^2 + 2AB\cos2\Theta$
 $C^2 = (4)^2 + (1.75)^2 + 2(4)(1.75)\cos110$
 $C^2 = 16 + 3.0625 + (14)(-0.34202)$
 $C^2 = 14.27422$
 $C = 3.778$, or approximately 3.75

This is the resultant cylinder power.

2. $\sin2\phi = \dfrac{B}{C} \sin2\Theta$

$\sin2\phi = \dfrac{1.75}{3.778} (0.93969)$

$\sin2\phi = (0.463208)(0.93969)$

$\sin2\phi = 0.43527$

$2\phi = 25.80247$

$\phi = 12.901235°$, or $12°54'4.45''$

This is the angular amount to be added to the A axis to obtain the resultant axis.

$80° + 12°54'4.45'' = 92°54'4.45''$

Therefore, the resultant axis is approximately 93 degrees.

3. $S = \dfrac{A + B - C}{2}$

$S = \dfrac{4 + 1.75 - 3.778}{2}$

$S = 0.986$

This is the amount to be added to the other sphere power.

Pl $+ 1.00 + 0.986 = 1.986$

The resultant sphere power is approximately 2.00.

If you add Pl $+4.00 \times 80$ and $+1.00 +1.75 \times 135$, the resultant prescription will be $+2.00 +3.75 \times 93$.

Chapter 18.
Executive and
Progressive Multifocals

Executive and progressive multifocals require some unique fabricating adjustments due to the construction of the near point or addition on these one-piece lenses. The executive style provides the most visible example of this near point construction. This style appears to be two lenses—one for distance and one for near vision—glued together, forming a straight line at their intersection. This, however, is not the case. It is really one lens with two distinctly different curves ground on the same surface. The difference between the two curves is the add power. For example, if a lens has a +6.00D curve on the distance portion with a +8.00D curve on the near portion, the add is +2.00D.

Each manufacturer of progressive lenses has its own design. However, if we consider progressive lenses in the simplest of terms, they are all alike. Their purpose is to gradually steepen the near point curve. This eliminates the distinct line between the distance and near, and, because it graduates the curve, it creates a variety of adds or focal lengths. As the wearer glances down through the various adds, this "trombone" effect creates adequate vision at several distances. The basic differences between progressive lenses lie in the amount of horizontal and vertical space used for this change, as well as the shape and horizontal and vertical size of the full add.

Thickness Compensation

The first place an adjustment must be made is in figuring the shop slip. The lens thickness must be calculated with the curve change in mind. Go back to thinking of the executive-style lens as two separate lenses. The bottom lens containing the near correction has more plus power than the top lens. We know that the higher the plus power, the thicker a lens must be to retain the desired diameter. Therefore, we must consider the total power at near when computing the needed thickness to avoid making too small a lens. The inside curve is calculated normally, using the distance prescription, because the power difference is created by the differing outside curves.

Progressive lenses do not require as much thickness compensation as the executive style, because the total add plus power does not go completely across the bottom of the lens. The substantial variations in segment size and design require that you follow the manufacturer's specifications exactly. Some labs have successfully readapted their computers' executive-style program for progressives. With some experimentation you may find that your executive-style program will work if you feed in a reduced add power. A place to start your experimentation would be at one-half the add power. There are also newer computers programmed to handle many of the progressive styles without any adaptation necessary.

Blocking

The next place an adjustment must be made is in the blocking procedure. The multifront curve style of a multifocal does not present a level blocking surface, so the lens will rock on the blocking ring. To avoid unwanted prism, these lenses must be blocked with pressure down on the distance portion only. This will seal the distance portion down to the blocking ring. You can expect the alloy to leak out the near portion of the lens.

Some manufacturers have designed special executive-style blocking molds, which also form an alloy generator sphere ring to aid in chucking. The larger Coburn aluminum blocks designed for plastic lenses also work very well and use less alloy. The basic difference between these two methods appears at the generator. Generating prism using the executive-style mold requires prism wedges, while standard prism rings can be used on the plastic-style block. This may not make much difference to you, but be aware of the two possible problems:

1. Unwanted cross prism is more easily induced using prism wedges.
2. If you mark the prism on the lens at its base, your prism rings are marked at their apex. This means that the prism direction must be reversed when using prism wedges, because a prism wedge makes the apex of the prism in the lens. It is foolish to artificially create possible problems by overcomplicating your system in this manner.

All of these adjustments must be considered when working with any executive- or progressive-style multifocal. In addition, most progressive styles have individually distinctive procedures that must be followed. Thoroughly familiarize yourself with the manufacturer's specifications before you begin fabrication.

Locating Optical Center

The correct location of the executive-style multifocal's near OC with respect to the distance OC has been a long-standing controversy.

Case 1

First let us examine the following case: Due to the frame size and needed decentration, the lens cuts out easily, with the OC in the horizontal center of the blank. This is the same as saying a finished single-vision blank would cut out; the only difference is that a finished single-vision lens already has the OC located in the center of the blank. With the executive-style multifocal you must locate two OCs in portions of the lens having two different powers.

In our first example, no prism needs to be ground. All we have to do is grind the OC on center, and the finished blank can be decentered over to obtain the correct PD. Unfortunately, this will only achieve one of the PDs. When you grind without prism, the distance and near OCs will be decentered identically. Wherever you block the lens, the OCs will appear. You can obtain decentration by moving your blocking center over, but you cannot create a horizontal difference between the OCs. Therefore, the distance and near PDs will be the same on the finished pair of glasses.

The question arises, For which PD should the lens be decentered? Unless the doctor specifies otherwise, the decentration is generally figured for the distance PD, the theory being that the decentration should be correct through the most-used portion of the lens. However, do not be surprised if the doctor asks you to split the difference or use the near PD as your reference. This could be based on what the patient is now wearing, the need to induce prism, or other factors.

Case 2

There may be no possible way to decenter the lens far enough to obtain the PD if the OCs are ground on center. It is then necessary to relocate the OC nasally on the blank to obtain cutout and PD. One way to do this is as previously mentioned, using off-center blocking. Remember to add the decentration amount into your thickness calculations. This method generally is not used because it can create fabricating problems. On-center blocking makes the fabricating process much easier.

The only other way to relocate the OC on a lens is to grind prism just as we did on a semifinished single-vision blank. The only problem is that an executive-style multifocal is more like two different single-vision lenses. Therefore, the amount of prism necessary to move over the distance OC correctly will not move over the near OC correctly.

Some Examples

Let us look at some examples. Assume that it is necessary to move the OC nasally 5mm.

In our first example, consider the prescription -3.00 sphere with a $+1.00$ add. The power in the distance is -3.00, and the power at near is -2.00. If you wish to move the OC in the -3.00 area 5mm, you must grind 1.5Δ base out:

$$-3 \times 0.5 = -1.5\Delta$$

Since you are not grinding the prism in the distance only, the near OC will also be moved.

$$-2 \times \frac{d}{10} = -1.5\Delta$$
$$d = 7.5mm$$

As you can see, the near OC will move in 2.5mm more than the distance OC. This is approximately 1mm more per eye than you would want to obtain a good distance-to-near relationship. This is certainly nothing to be upset about with this lens style.

In our second example, consider the prescription +3.00 sphere with a +2.00 add. The power in the distance is +3.00, and the power at near is +5.00. If you wish to move the OC in the +3.00 area 5mm, you must grind 1.5Δ base in:

$$+3 \times 0.5 = 1.5\Delta$$

Unfortunately, the near OC will not be affected as nicely as it was in the first example:

$$+5 \times \frac{d}{10} = 1.5\Delta$$
$$d = 3mm$$

In this case the near OC moved in 2mm less than the distance OC. If the patient's PD were 66/63, you would end up with 66/70, or a 7mm near error. This certainly is not a satisfactory pair of glasses. If you must obtain the distance or near OC, the best you can do is use as much of the blank as possible for decentration and grind prism for the balance of the decentration. You will simply have to let the OC not decentered for, go wherever the prism pushes it. Because of this problem, most labs use specific policies when grinding their executive-style multifocals unless otherwise specified by the account.

As our third example, consider the prescription −1.00 sphere with a +2.00 add. The power in the distance is −1.00, and the power at near is +1.00. If you wish to move the OC in the −1.00 area 5mm, you must grind 0.5Δ base out:

$$-1 \times 0.5 = -0.5\Delta$$

Now comes the real problem. Grinding base out prism on this lens will not only move the near OC an incorrect amount; it will move it the wrong way:

$$+1 \times \frac{d}{10} = -0.5\Delta$$
$$d = -5mm$$

That minus sign in front of the 5mm means that the near OC will be moving temporally 5mm. At the same time, the distance OC moved nasally 5mm. That is a 10mm difference. When seeking a 66/63 PD you would end up with a 66/86 PD. This is the ultimate in poor optics. You would have been farther ahead to have offset blocked without prism and have perhaps obtained a 70/70 PD.

Blank Size

It is possible to use this characteristic of variable OC movement to create the perfect lens. Some computer programs will calculate the amount of prism necessary to create the inset you wish. We almost did just that in the first example. The only problem generally is in the blank size. The amount of prism necessary to create the desired inset may locate the OCs where the total decentration cannot be achieved due to cutout. In other words, you may be seeking a 66/63 PD and obtain a 73/70 PD. The inset is correct, but you ran out of lens for decentration.

In the second example we had a $+3.00$ sphere distance with a $+5.00$ near power. Do not concern yourself with the decentration necessary to obtain cutout. Instead, we will obtain the 1.5mm inset required if a patient's PD were 66/63. You will notice that the near, having more power, was affected less by the prism than the distance. There is no way to grind base in prism on this lens and have the near OC move farther in nasally than the distance OC.

But what would happen if you ground base out prism instead? The distance OC, having less power, would move temporally at a faster rate than the near OC. Therefore, by grinding prism the wrong way, you can obtain a near inset. If you grind 1.2Δ base out, the distance OC will move temporally 4mm:

$$+3 \times \frac{d}{10} = -1.2\Delta$$
$$d = -4.0mm$$

The same 1.2Δ base out will only move the near OC temporally 2.4mm:

$$+5 \times \frac{d}{10} = -1.2\Delta$$
$$d = -2.4$$

Therefore, the near OC is 1.6mm nearer the nasal edge of the lens than the distance OC, and the inset has been created (4 − 2.4 = 1.6).

The only possible problem with this method is if you do not have enough lens blank to physically move the lens to obtain the decentration after having moved the distance OC 4mm the wrong way. If, as in the second example, we needed 5mm of decentration via prism, we would be off not only that 5mm, but also the 4mm of decentration the wrong way. The inset would be correct, but the PD would be off 9mm per eye.

Do not be misled by this example; this method will work in some cases. There is a variety of ways to control the OC, and eventual distance and near PD with executive-style multifocals. The restrictions are caused more by the available blank sizes than anything else. In plastic lenses there are larger blank sizes that are much more applicable to various OC control methods than in the case of glass lenses. There are even blanks available with predecentered near OCs. This is certainly of assistance with some of the grinding techniques discussed here.

Chapter 19.
Round and
Blended Multifocals

Most blended multifocals are nothing more than round segs with their outer edges blended to remove the sharp line of transition from distance to near caused by the two different indexes of refraction used in a glass lens. In plastic lenses this line is caused by the two different curves used.

Segment Variations

Realistically, a sharp line of demarcation between the distance and near prescriptions is optically sounder and generally easier for the wearer to adapt to. However, with vanity and aesthetics comes the desire to hide the multifocal line that many people incorrectly associate with old age. People are willing to adapt to a larger area of distance-to-near transition that is of no optical use to partially hide the multifocal.

The dispenser is faced with an interesting problem. There are many blended multifocals on the market. The difference between them is basically how large the usable seg is, how well the seg is hidden and how large the transition area is. Basically, the better the seg is hidden, the larger the blended or transition area must be. The usable seg size does not have to be small to have a good blend. If the manufacturer were to start with a very large seg, the lens could still have a large usable seg even after a substantial transition area was created. Unfortunately, many manufacturers are starting with a standard-sized seg. Once they blend into this size seg, only a relatively small usable seg is left.

The dispenser must be concerned with the patient's needs. How large a reading area is needed? How well must the seg be hidden? How adaptable is the patient to a blended area? These questions plus many more must be answered before selecting which, if any, blended multifocal can be used by the patient. In the lab we are not responsible for this decision. However, knowing the manufacturers' differences will be helpful during fabrication.

Markup

The only fabrication step that differs between round-style and flat top segs is lens markup. Flat top multifocals can be decentered for the seg inset only, and to avoid a crooked seg line they must not be twisted. A round seg can be twisted in to accommodate the total decentration prior to decentering for the seg inset. This is almost as though you can locate the seg any place on the blank to achieve cutout.

First, calculate the distance decentration per eye. This is the amount the seg will be twisted in. Place the lens blank on the center of your protractor or marker, and then twist it in. With the convex side facing up toward you, a counterclockwise rotation would create a right lens and a clockwise rotation a left lens. When you twist the seg in, you must not change the position of the blank on the protractor; the blank must remain on center. Twist the blank as though it turned around its center like a record, without moving up or down— only around.

Next, calculate the seg drop in the same manner as with any multifocal, and locate the seg accordingly. When you move the lens blank up or down to properly locate the seg, the lens must not be twisted or moved horizontally. Imagine that after the first step you created a flat top multifocal with the seg located where needed in the blank. In the second step you created the seg, drop as you would have with any flat top multifocal.

In the third and last step you must create the seg inset, then mark the lens at the appropriate axis. Since the initial rotation in step one, you have probably moved the seg out quite a bit more than what the inset should be. You therefore must slide the seg back toward the center of the marker. Do not twist or move the lens vertically while sliding the lens back horizontally. Just think what it would do to a flat top seg if the lens were twisted or moved vertically. Once you have moved the lens back to create the inset, all that is left is to mark the axis and prism at that point. (See Figure 23.)

When working with a blended seg, make a round seg out of it by outlining with a marker the blended portion where it meets the distance prescription. Some people also mark the center of the seg for a point of reference. You may find it even easier if you mark a regular round seg.

Suggestions for Fabrication

If the necessary rotation is excessive, you could find yourself blocking the lens in a very bad place for fabrication. It is possible to move the blocking center over to the horizontal center of the blank for fabricating ease. The amount the blocking center is moved times the power through the 180-degree meridian will give you the amount of prism necessary to grind the optical center back over to where it belongs. You may similarly make a vertical blocking center adjustment to compensate for a difficult seg drop location. This would be accomplished by calculating the blocking center movement times the power through the 90-degree meridian. If both movements are necessary, simply calculate the compound prism (see Figure 24).

When working with plus lenses, be careful that the on-center compensation does not create more of a problem than if you had not compensated to begin with. The two points to remember are (1) with lenses in general, the thickness is the same equidistant from the optical center; and (2) specifically with plus lenses, the diameter will be reduced as the center thickness decreases. Taking both of these points into consideration, the center of the blank will probably not turn out to be the center of the generated lens. You may end up grinding prism so that you are blocking the lens in the center of the blank, only to find out that you will be blocked way off center of the generated lens.

Chapter 20.
Slab-Off Grinding

By inspecting a cross section of a plus and minus lens, you can discover an interesting trait: The lenses appear to be constructed of prisms. A plus lens appears to be two prisms joined at their bases, and a minus lens two prisms joined at their apexes.

Prismatic Effect

The curves on a lens magnify or minify. While doing so, however, they create the same prismatic effect as a standard prism. The strength of a prism is measured in its rise or thickness difference between the apex and base. Therefore, you can see that the greater the magnifying or minifying power of a lens, the greater its prismatic effect.

Power-to-Prism Formula

Consider the standard power-to-prism formula for both glass and plastic lenses:

$$\Delta = \frac{P \times D}{10}$$

The prism equals the power of the lens times the amount of decentration (in millimeters) divided by ten.

The formula shows that the greater the deviation (decentration) from the point where the prism has no effect, the stronger the prismatic effect becomes. The point of no prismatic effect is where the prisms meet. In a plus lens this is where the bases meet, and in a minus lens it is where the apexes meet. This point, where rays of light are not bent, is the optical center.

Now you can see why it is so important to decenter the OC directly over the pupil. Any other portion of the lens over the pupil will create a prismatic effect. The amount of effect is measured using the formula above: the amount of power through the meridian where the error is times the distance the OC is off divided by ten. Everything is just fine as long as a person looks through the OC. But what happens when the eyes glance away? The brain has the unique ability to temporarily compensate for some of the prismatic effect created when the eyes glance around. A problem arises when they spend too much time in an area of the lens that produces more prism than the brain can compensate for. This generally occurs in glancing down to read. From the eyeglass wearer's point of view, prism displaces or moves images. When the wearer glances down to read, the image is displaced by each eye. If the image is displaced up or down an equal amount in each eye, the brain has no trouble adapting. If the power is not the same, an unequal amount of displacement will occur. The amount of prism-induced image displacement people are able to compensate for varies from patient to patient.

This creates a point of disagreement among practitioners. Once a patient proves unable to compensate for the image displacement, should they neutralize the image displacement totally, or just enough so the patient can compensate the balance? This can create a fabricating problem. What do you do when the account gives you an amount of compensation that will not totally neutralize the displacement? Is the account allowing the patient to do some compensating, or did the account miscalculate? This is another time that it would be very nice to have a working relationship with your accounts. Most labs ignore the account's request and simply calculate the amount of compensation necessary to totally neutralize the entire displacement. These labs arrive at this decision to avoid a run-in with the account. Some accounts take offense at being questioned. What a price for pride! The patient may suffer.

Neutralizing Image Displacement

What must be done to compensate for this image displacement? The only way to neutralize prism is with another prism of the same power but of opposite direction or base. The prismatic problem occurs on only part of the lens. The neutralizing prism, therefore, must appear only on that part of the lens. We must calculate the amount and location of the neutralizing prism.

This prism is called a *slab-off prism* or simply a *slab*. The prism is ground from the top of the lens down to the top of the segment line. In a single-vision lens the prism is ground from the top of the lens down to the account's requested height. You do not see as many slabs on single-vision lenses as on multifocals, because the wearers can merely lower their heads until they are looking through the optical centers to eliminate the displacement at near. Multifocal wearers do not have that option, since they must glance down to look through their near correction. The amount of prism necessary to neutralize the displacement can be calculated easily using the standard power-to-prism formula. The two variables that are needed for the formula are power and decentration.

Power

The amount of power we are concerned with runs through the 90-degree meridian. If you do not have a sphere, it will be necessary to calculate how much the cylinder will affect the sphere through the 90-degree meridian. The formula for that is the following:

$$P = C \times \cos^2 A$$

The power or effect the cylinder will have on the sphere equals the amount of cylinder times the cosine squared of the angle of the cylinder. There are charts for this, but let us look at an example of how the formula works. What is the power through the 90-degree meridian in the prescription $-4.00 \; -3.00 \times 65$?

$$P = C \times \cos^2 A$$
$$P = -3 \times \cos^2 65$$
$$P = -0.537$$

Remember, this is the amount that the cylinder affects the sphere power through the 90-degree meridian. Combine the sphere power with the cylinder effect to determine the power through the 90-degree meridian.

$$-4.00 + (-0.537) = -4.537$$

You must find how much power runs through the 90-degree meridian of both the right and left lenses. The difference in power between the two eyes causes the image displacement. Calculate the difference between the 90-degree meridian powers, and use this difference in the power-to-prism formula.

Decentration

The other variable in the formula is decentration. In this context, decentration is the distance from the near OC up to the distance OC. The location of the near OC in the segment can vary depending on the lens manufacturer. For our example we will assume that the near OC is 5mm below the top of the seg line in a D-25. In all glasses the distance OC is ground at one-half the B dimension of the lens.

Calculate as you would for any multifocal layout. If the seg turns out to be 4mm below, you know that the distance from the top of the seg line up to the distance OC is 4mm. We previously stated that the near OC was 5mm below the seg line. Therefore, the distance between the distance and near OCs would be 9mm in this case. This 9mm times the 90-degree meridian power difference divided by ten is the amount of prism needed to neutralize the image displacement. With respect to the top of the seg line, the prism will need to be base up. Since you are grinding the prism from the top of the lens down to the seg line, it will need to be base down prism with respect to the entire lens surface.

As you can see, the calculation is very simple. All you need to know is the power difference between the right and the left lens through the 90-degree meridian and the distance the eye will glance down to read. By applying these two numbers in the power-to-prism formula, you will obtain the needed prism. Always grind the prism on the most minus or least plus lens. By grinding base down prism from the top of the lens down to the top of the seg line, you will create base up prism at near.

Evaluation

There are two basic flaws in this standard method for slab calculation. When this method was developed years ago, eyeglasses were fit with the patient's pupil at one-half the B measurement. If this is not the case, the calculations cannot be correct. If any pair of glasses is to be really correct, we must know a pupil height with respect to the B dimension of the lens. After all, that is what a PD is for. We work so hard to eliminate horizontal prism and totally ignore vertical prism. Our concern seems to be the elimination of vertical prism at one-half B, regardless of how much a problem this may create for the patient. Even single-vision lenses should be prescribed with a pupil height.

This is a basic prescribing flaw and certainly not the lab's problem. You should understand the problem, however, because this is an area that could create patient discomfort with new glasses. When the account tells you that a patient cannot wear new glasses and neither you or the account can find anything wrong with them, consider vertical prism. Did the power through the 90-degree meridian change? Or is it possible that the new frame creates a poor or different pupil-to-one-half-B-location relationship? Now you find yourself grinding a slab for the sole purpose of eliminating vertical prism at near, and you do not even have the correct information. The odds of the slab being correct are very poor unless the frame fits correctly or a pupil height is given. It is no wonder that so many accounts have poor "luck" with slabs. The only change that should be made is to substitute the height of the pupil for one-half B. The distance or decentration in the formula will be from the pupil down to the near OC.

Eye-Level Differences

The second flaw is related to pupil height measurement. The fitting of progressive lenses created the need for taking more accurate measurements of pupil location. Every lab suddenly started receiving many more split seg heights. That is, the eyes are not sitting on the same level or at equidistant heights with respect to the frame.

When this eye-level difference exists, you must adjust the method of calculation. Calculate the prism difference per eye rather than the power difference. For each eye independently, calculate the amount of power running through the 90-degree meridian. Then, using the individual pupil-to-near-OC distances, establish the amount of prism in each eye. The difference between the right and left eye prism amounts is the amount of prism needed to neutralize the near vertical prism. As an example, how much slab-off prism would be needed to neutralize the following prescription?

$$OD \quad -2.00 \; -3.00 \times 170$$
$$OS \quad -1.00 \; -2.00 \times 80$$

Where 1. D-25, Right 14mm high, Left 13mm high.
           2. B dimension 40mm ($\frac{1}{2}$B = 20).
           3. Pupil height: Right 23mm, Left 21mm.

First, calculate the amount of power running through the 90-degree meridian of each eye.

$$\text{Right:} \quad P = C \cos^2 A$$
$$P = -3 \cos^2 170$$
$$P = -2.91$$
$$-2.91 + (-2.00) = -4.91$$
$$\text{Left:} \quad P = C \cos^2 A$$
$$P = -2 \cos^2 80$$
$$P = -0.06$$
$$-0.06 + (-1.00) = -1.06$$

Second, calculate the distance or decentration per eye:

Right: The seg height is 14mm high, or $20 - 14 = 6$mm below.
         The pupil height is 23mm high, or $23 - 20 = 3$mm above.
         The total distance is $6 + 3 = 9$mm.

Left: The seg height is 13mm high, or $20 - 13 = 7$mm below.
         The pupil height is 21mm high, or $21 - 20 = 1$mm above.
         The total distance is $7 + 1 = 8$mm.

Third, using the power-to-prism formula, calculate the amount of prism per eye:

$$\text{Right:} \; \Delta = \frac{P \times D}{10}$$
$$\Delta = \frac{-4.91 \times 9}{10}$$
$$\Delta = -4.419$$
$$\text{Left:} \; \Delta = \frac{P \times D}{10}$$
$$\Delta = \frac{-1.06 \times 8}{10}$$
$$\Delta = -0.848$$

Fourth, calculate the difference between the two prism amounts:

$$-4.419 - (-0.848) = -3.571$$

The correct answer is 3.5^Δ base down on the right eye.

It is highly unlikely that you will find many slabs with this many differences between the right and left eyes. However, you can see that by calculating your slabs in this manner, you have the opportunity to compensate for any differences. The four simple steps in calculating slab-off prism are summarized:

1. Calculate the amount of power through the 90-degree meridian of each eye.
2. Calculate the decentration per eye.
3. Calculate the amount of prism per eye.
4. Calculate the amount of prism difference.

Fabrication

The slab calculations just demonstrated are the same for both glass and plastic lenses. It is in fabrication that different procedures must be employed. Starting with glass, we will examine each procedure separately.

Let us review what we are attempting to accomplish. Due to a power difference between the right and left lenses, an image displacement occurs at the reading level. We can neutralize the displacement by creating base up prism in the reading area of the most minus or least plus lens. If we ground a base up prism on the plus side of a multifocal, the segment would be destroyed. Our only other option is to grind a base down prism from the top of the lens down to the seg line. This, will, in effect, create base up prism in the reading area. Most labs use basically the same method to accomplish this. The only major variable is whether we should grind the slab on the plus side first and then finish the minus side, or if we should reverse the order and do the inside first and then the plus side slab. We will review the procedure for slabbing the plus side first and then finishing the minus side.

Slabbing Plus Side (Glass)

Prepare the multifocal to be slabbed. Block on the plus side and zero cut the minus side of the multifocal until the curve is completely across the lens. This will remove any minus side prism from the lens manufacturer. Use approximately the same curve as was on the lens. Complete the lens by fining and polishing.

Prepare a cover lens. This lens, which will be attached to the front surface of the multifocal, serves two functions. First, it protects the area of the multifocal that is not going to be surfaced. Second, it serves as a guide as the slab line is moved down the lens. For the cover lens to adhere adequately to the plus side of the multifocal, the curves must be exact. Carefully sag and establish the multifocal's front curve. Block the cover lens on the plus side, and cut the minus side to match the multifocal's front curve. Some labs leave the cover lens unpolished as an aid in the adhering process. If the curve is cut adequately, this should not be necessary. Being able to see through the polished cover lens can be an advantage as the slab line approaches the seg.

Now attach the lenses together with balsam. Heat both the cover lens and the multifocal in an oven. (The oven used to bake plastic lenses will work very well.) When the two lenses have been completely heated to the 200°F. oven temperature, the balsam may be applied. Rub the balsam directly onto the plus surface of the multifocal and the matching inside surface of the cover lens. Use a thin but complete coating on both surfaces. Put the two lenses together, carefully pressing out the bubbles. Use pressure to force the bubbles out and hold the lenses together until they cool. Weight or the careful use of a wood clamp will work. Watch your fingers; use a towel or gloves to handle the lenses, because they are very hot. Cooling time is approximately one-half hour.

Prepare and block the lens. On the minus side you may wish to mark a 180-degree line across the lens at the seg height. If you are not using a polished cover lens, mark at least one other 180-degree line halfway down to the the seg line. Use that line to guide you toward a straight slab line before you reach the seg line. If the slab line is crooked, once you reach the seg it will be too late to do anything about it. Precoat and block in a normal manner on the minus surface of the multifocal. The block should be on center horizontally and either on center or slightly high vertically.

Generate the correct amount of base down prism. Bring the slab line down slowly by removing small amounts of glass at a time. The higher the amount of prism being ground, the nearer the seg line down to which you can generate the slab line. The slab line can come within 5mm of the seg on a very high prism. How near you can come to the seg depends on the amount of prism being ground and your ability.

The lens is now ready to be fined. How close the slab line is fined down to the seg depends on the same factors as in generating, and knowledge will come with experience. Stop the fining often to inspect the line for straightness. If the line is higher on one side than the other, offset fine on the high side until the line straightens. If both sides of the line are either higher or lower than the center of the line, the tool curve is either flatter or steeper than the lens curve. The tool must be trued more accurately.

You may also wish to check the accuracy of the prism while fining. This can be done two ways: with calipers using the chart on thickness difference for sharp-edged prisms (see Section III), or with a lens clock. To use a lens clock, part of the cover lens would have had to be removed prior to attachment to the multifocal. Reduce the size of the cover lens approximately 5mm by flattening one side only. When the cover lens is attached to the multifocal, allow an area of noncovered multifocal to appear at the nasal side of the multifocal. This is the area most likely to cut out in case a problem is created by not covering the multifocal. This opening is used for the lens clock. With the lens clock, measure the curve of the slabbed area. Then, with the middle point of the lens clock directly on the slab line, one point in the slabbed area, and one point in the unslabbed area, take another curvature reading. The difference between the two curvature readings is the amount of prism. When you are happy with the straightness of the slab line, its closeness to the seg, and the amount of prism, you are ready to polish the lens.

Some labs use two separate tools: one for fining and one for polishing. They will generally use a hard pitch pad for polishing, and generally this method will give the sharpest, most distinct slab line. Again, check the straightness of the slab line to assure the proper tool curve. Some labs have had success using a one-tool method and their standard cylinder-style polishing pads. This may work for you, depending on the type of pad and machinery used.

Deblock but do not remove the cover lens. The slabbed lens may now be treated like any other multifocal. Mark, block, and run the inside curve normally.

Deblock and clean the lens. The cover lens may be removed by reheating the lens in the oven. When the lens is warm enough, slide off the cover plate with a pencil eraser. Residual balsam may be removed with acetone after cooling.

Inspect the lens. The slab amount can be checked with a lens clock, as discussed earlier. If you were to nullify all the vertical image displacement, a Lensometer is the best way to inspect the results. Neutralize the lens for the nonslabbed eye in the seg. At approximately 5mm below the seg line, note the amount of vertical prism present, and spot the seg. Neutralize the slabbed lens in the seg. Move the lens vertically until you create the same amount of prism present in the non-slabbed lens, and spot the seg. If the spots in the slabbed and nonslabbed segs are the same distance below the seg line, the vertical prism between the lenses has been neutralized. If the spots are not the same distance below the seg line, reneutralize the slabbed lens. This time, move the lens the direction needed to match the other lens until you reach the vertical prism tolerance, and respot. If the spots are now the same distance or the slab spot has gone farther than necessary, you are within tolerance.

Slabbing Minus Side (Plastic)

Plastic slabs are fabricated differently than glass slabs: A plastic slab is put on the minus side of the lens rather than the plus side, mainly because it would be difficult to work around the raised segment.

The fact that the slab is ground on the minus side has led to some very diverse opinions on how the prism should be ground. Remember, we want to create base up prism on the most minus or least plus lens with respect to the top of the seg line. In glass we had to grind base down prism from the top of the lens to the seg line to create base up prism at near. The reason for this was that if we ground base up prism from the bottom of the lens up to the seg line, we would destroy the seg.

With plastic, we are grinding the slab on the minus side, so there is no reason not to grind the prism base up from the bottom of the lens up to the seg line. There also is no reason not to grind the prism base down from the top of the lens down to the seg. One way is not any better than the other; each has advantages and disadvantages. When the slab line is brought from the bottom up, the already surfaced distance portion is covered and protected. If the slab line is brought from the top down, the distance portion is surfaced twice. Some labs would rather not take that chance with the distance portion. They would prefer to surface the near portion of the lens twice. The distance from the top of the lens down to the seg line is much greater than the distance from the bottom of the lens up to the seg line. This is a disadvantage, because the slab line must be held straight longer. It is also an advantage, especially on low-powered slabs; it gives you more room to correct prism amounts and slab line straightness.

Experiment and discover the best method for you. An example incorporates both of these methods into one. The slab and the needed curve will be cut all at once. Therefore, mark the lens not only with the normal layout marks, but also with a 180-degree line across the line at the seg height. Block the lens normally.

When you first generate the lens, cut the needed inside curve and the needed prism for the slab at the same time. The prism will go across the entire surface of the lens. You must grind base up prism—not base down. By cutting the prism all the way across the lens, you may more easily caliper the amount of prism. This is the most accurate way to check the prism and eliminate cross prism when grinding a slab. Check the accuracy of the slab prism just like you would any other prism.

Fine and polish the lens normally. Do not deblock the lens.

Now create a cover lens for the inside curve. It would be too much work to make an actual lens to use as a cover, because the inside curve probably is not a sphere. Attaching the lens would be another problem. Instead, make a perfectly curved matched lens by pouring "liquid lens" into the minus curve of the lens. Once it hardens it will perfectly match and be securely attached to the lens. This "liquid lens" can be made out of many different substances. Labs generally use plastic resin, epoxy, or even cold-blocking compound. Use a clear precoat on the minus side of the lens. Mix the resin according to the instructions on the product being used. Pour a thin covering of the resin over the entire surface. It is not necessary to pool the resin up on the half of the lens that will not be ground away (the bottom half in this case). You may wish to use tape around the lens to form a mold and prevent overflow. However, many labs that use tape end up filling the mold. This uses too much resin. As these resins set up, they create substantial heat. The more resin used, the more heat will be created. Remember, heat is an enemy to a plastic lens. Not only could you ruin the lens; it may even deblock at an inopportune time from heat stress. Allow the resin to set up properly overnight.

The lens now should be regenerated with the same needed curve, but this time without the prism. A slab line will appear at the top of the lens and slowly move down toward the seg as more material is removed. The distance from the seg line you must stop depends on the amount of prism and your ability, just like in glass.

Fine the lens. Check the lens often for straightness of the line. Use finger pressure on the high line side while fining to straighten the line. The fining pad will have to be cleaned of lens cover resin often. When you stop the machine, check the slab line and clean the resin off the pad with a brush. When the slab line gets as close to the seg line as the amount of prism will allow, do a second fine. How close the slab line is to the seg after the first or second fine depends on the same factors as in generating and will come with experience. Again, check the line, and if necessary clean the pad. This will not be required as often as it was with the first fine pad. Stop second fining when you are as close to the seg line as the amount of prism will allow.

Polish the lens in a normal manner. Deblock the lens, and peel or lift the resin off with a knife. It may help to run hot water or immerse the lens in the reclaim tank first. Clean the lens with acetone.

A plastic slab may be inspected in the same manner as a glass slab. Use either the lens clock or Lensometer method.

Only small changes are necessary if you would prefer to bring the slab line up from the bottom of the lens to the seg line:

1. When you generate the lens the first time, cut only the needed curve. Do not grind the prism for the slab.

2. The second time you generate the lens, cut the needed curve again along with the prism for the slab. The prism must be base up.

3. Check the lens often while fining, because you do not have much room to correct the amount of prism or the straightness of the slab line.

With a little experimentation you may find that each method may be superior, depending on the prescription.

SECTION III

Charts

A. PERCENT OF CYLINDER POWER THROUGH 180 DEGREES

Angle in degrees	% of effect at 180°
0/180	0
5/175	0.008
10/170	0.030
15/165	0.067
20/160	0.117
25/155	0.179
30/150	0.250
35/145	0.329
40/140	0.413
45/135	0.500
50/130	0.587
55/125	0.671
60/120	0.750
65/115	0.821
70/110	0.883
75/105	0.933
80/100	0.970
85/95	0.992
90	1

$$P = \sin^2 A$$

The percent the cylinder will affect the sphere power at 180 degrees equals the sine squared of the cylinder angle.

To calculate how much a cylinder will affect the sphere power at 180 degrees, multiply the amount of cylinder times the percentage factor at its angle. For example, what is the power through the 180 degree meridian in the prescription $-4.00 \ -3.00 \times 65$?

$$-3 \times 0.821 \ = \ -2.463$$
$$-4.00 + (-2.463) \ = \ -6.463$$
through the 180 degree meridian

B. PERCENT OF CYLINDER POWER THROUGH 90 DEGREES

Angle in degrees	% of effect at 90°
0/180	1
5/175	0.992
10/170	0.970
15/165	0.933
20/160	0.883
25/155	0.821
30/150	0.750
35/145	0.671
40/140	0.587
45/135	0.500
50/130	0.413
55/125	0.329
60/120	0.250
65/115	0.179
70/110	0.117
75/105	0.067
80/100	0.030
85/95	0.008
90	0

$$P = \cos^2 A$$

The percent the cylinder power will affect the sphere power at 90 degrees equals the cosine squared of the cylinder angle.

To calculate how much a cylinder will affect the sphere power at 90 degrees, multiply the amount of cylinder times the percentage factor at its angle. For example, what is the power through the 90 degree meridian in the prescription $-4.00 \ -3.00 \times 65$?

$$-3 \times 0.179 \ = \ -0.537$$
$$-4.00 + (-0.537) \ = \ -4.537$$

through the 90 degree meridian

C. PLASTIC 1.498 COMPENSATION

Power	Comp.	Power	Comp.	Power	Comp.	Power	Comp.	Power	Comp.
0.12	0.128	4.12	4.385	8.12	8.642	12.12	12.899	16.12	17.156
0.25	0.266	4.25	4.523	8.25	8.780	12.25	13.037	16.25	17.294
0.37	0.394	4.37	4.651	8.37	8.908	12.37	13.165	16.37	17.422
0.50	0.532	4.50	4.789	8.50	9.046	12.50	13.303	16.50	17.560
0.62	0.660	4.62	4.917	8.62	9.174	12.62	13.431	16.62	17.688
0.75	0.798	4.75	5.055	8.75	9.312	12.75	13.569	16.75	17.826
0.87	0.926	4.87	5.183	8.87	9.440	12.87	13.697	16.87	17.954
1.00	1.064	5.00	5.321	9.00	9.578	13.00	13.835	17.00	18.092
1.12	1.192	5.12	5.449	9.12	9.706	13.12	13.963	17.12	18.220
1.25	1.330	5.25	5.587	9.25	9.844	13.25	14.101	17.25	18.358
1.37	1.458	5.37	5.715	9.37	9.972	13.37	14.229	17.37	18.486
1.50	1.596	5.50	5.853	9.50	10.110	13.50	14.367	17.50	18.624
1.62	1.724	5.62	5.981	9.62	10.238	13.62	14.495	17.62	18.752
1.75	1.862	5.75	6.119	9.75	10.377	13.75	14.634	17.75	18.891
1.87	1.990	5.87	6.247	9.87	10.504	13.87	14.761	17.87	19.018
2.00	2.129	6.00	6.386	10.00	10.643	14.00	14.900	18.00	19.157
2.12	2.256	6.12	6.513	10.12	10.770	14.12	15.027	18.12	19.284
2.25	2.395	6.25	6.652	10.25	10.909	14.25	15.166	18.25	19.423
2.37	2.522	6.37	6.779	10.37	11.036	14.37	15.293	18.37	19.550
2.50	2.661	6.50	6.918	10.50	11.175	14.50	15.432	18.50	19.689
2.62	2.788	6.62	7.045	10.62	11.302	14.62	15.560	18.62	19.816
2.75	2.927	6.75	7.184	10.75	11.441	14.75	15.698	18.75	19.955
2.87	3.054	6.87	7.311	10.87	11.568	14.87	15.826	18.87	20.083
3.00	3.193	7.00	7.450	11.00	11.707	15.00	15.964	19.00	20.221
3.12	3.320	7.12	7.578	11.12	11.835	15.12	16.092	19.12	20.349
3.25	3.459	7.25	7.716	11.25	11.973	15.25	16.230	19.25	20.487
3.37	3.587	7.37	7.844	11.37	12.101	15.37	16.358	19.37	20.615
3.50	3.725	7.50	7.982	11.50	12.239	15.50	16.496	19.50	20.753
3.62	3.853	7.62	8.110	11.62	12.367	15.62	16.624	19.62	20.881
3.75	3.991	7.75	8.248	11.75	12.505	15.75	16.762	19.75	21.019
3.87	4.119	7.87	8.376	11.87	12.633	15.87	16.890	19.87	21.147
4.00	4.257	8.00	8.514	12.00	12.771	16.00	17.028	20.00	21.285

The second column (compensation) gives the amount of power or curve in 1.498 index material necessary to achieve the power in the first column. The basis for the first column is traditionally 1.530 index.

The compensation factor is calculated by the following formula:

$$\frac{1.530 - 1}{1.498 - 1} = 1.064257028$$

For example, what power must you grind in 1.498 index material if the requested prescription power is −9.00?

$$1.064257028 \times -9 = -9.57831325$$

D. GLASS 1.523 COMPENSATION

Power	Comp.	Power	Comp.	Power	Comp.	Power	Comp.	Power	Comp.
0.12	0.121	4.12	4.175	8.12	8.229	12.12	12.282	16.12	16.336
0.25	0.253	4.25	4.307	8.25	8.360	12.25	12.414	16.25	16.467
0.37	0.375	4.37	4.428	8.37	8.482	12.37	12.536	16.37	16.589
0.50	0.507	4.50	4.560	8.50	8.614	12.50	12.667	16.50	16.721
0.62	0.628	4.62	4.682	8.62	8.735	12.62	12.789	16.62	16.842
0.75	0.760	4.75	4.814	8.75	8.867	12.75	12.921	16.75	16.974
0.87	0.882	4.87	4.935	8.87	8.989	12.87	13.042	16.87	17.096
1.00	1.013	5.00	5.067	9.00	9.120	13.00	13.174	17.00	17.228
1.12	1.135	5.12	5.189	9.12	9.242	13.12	13.296	17.12	17.349
1.25	1.267	5.25	5.320	9.25	9.374	13.25	13.427	17.25	17.481
1.37	1.388	5.37	5.442	9.37	9.495	13.37	13.549	17.37	17.602
1.50	1.520	5.50	5.574	9.50	9.627	13.50	13.681	17.50	17.734
1.62	1.642	5.62	5.695	9.62	9.749	13.62	13.802	17.62	17.856
1.75	1.773	5.75	5.827	9.75	9.880	13.75	13.934	17.75	17.988
1.87	1.895	5.87	5.949	9.87	10.002	13.87	14.056	17.87	18.109
2.00	2.027	6.00	6.080	10.00	10.134	14.00	14.187	18.00	18.241
2.12	2.148	6.12	6.202	10.12	10.255	14.12	14.309	18.12	18.363
2.25	2.280	6.25	6.334	10.25	10.387	14.25	14.441	18.25	18.494
2.37	2.402	6.37	6.455	10.37	10.509	14.37	14.562	18.37	18.616
2.50	2.533	6.50	6.587	10.50	10.641	14.50	14.694	18.50	18.748
2.62	2.655	6.62	6.709	10.62	10.762	14.62	14.816	18.62	18.869
2.75	2.787	6.75	6.840	10.75	10.894	14.75	14.947	18.75	19.001
2.87	2.908	6.87	6.962	10.87	11.015	14.87	15.069	18.87	19.123
3.00	3.040	7.00	7.094	11.00	11.147	15.00	15.200	19.00	19.254
3.12	3.162	7.12	7.215	11.12	11.269	15.12	15.322	19.12	19.376
3.25	3.293	7.25	7.347	11.25	11.401	15.25	15.454	19.25	19.508
3.37	3.415	7.37	7.469	11.37	11.522	15.37	15.576	19.37	19.629
3.50	3.547	7.50	7.600	11.50	11.654	15.50	15.707	19.50	19.761
3.62	3.668	7.62	7.722	11.62	11.776	15.62	15.829	19.62	19.883
3.75	3.800	7.75	7.854	11.75	11.907	15.75	15.961	19.75	20.014
3.87	3.922	7.87	7.975	11.87	12.029	15.87	16.082	19.87	20.136
4.00	4.054	8.00	8.107	12.00	12.161	16.00	16.214	20.00	20.268

The second column (compensation) gives the amount of power or curve in 1.523 index material necessary to achieve the power in the first column. The basis for the first column is traditionally 1.530 index.

The compensation factor is calculated by the following formula:

$$\frac{1.530 - 1}{1.523 - 1} = 1.013384321$$

For example, what power must you grind in 1.523 index material if the requested prescription power is −9.00?

$$1.013384321 \times -9 = -9.12045889$$

E.   GLASS 1.7 COMPENSATION

Power	Comp.	Power	Comp.	Power	Comp.	Power	Comp.	Power	Comp.
0.12	0.091	4.12	3.119	8.12	6.148	12.12	9.177	16.12	12.205
0.25	0.189	4.25	3.218	8.25	6.246	12.25	9.275	16.25	12.304
0.37	0.280	4.37	3.309	8.37	6.337	12.37	9.366	16.37	12.394
0.50	0.379	4.50	3.407	8.50	6.436	12.50	9.464	16.50	12.493
0.62	0.469	4.62	3.498	8.62	6.527	12.62	9.555	16.62	12.584
0.75	0.568	4.75	3.596	8.75	6.625	12.75	9.654	16.75	12.682
0.87	0.659	4.87	3.687	8.87	6.716	12.87	9.744	16.87	12.773
1.00	0.757	5.00	3.786	9.00	6.814	13.00	9.843	17.00	12.871
1.12	0.848	5.12	3.877	9.12	6.905	13.12	9.934	17.12	12.962
1.25	0.946	5.25	3.975	9.25	7.004	13.25	10.032	17.25	13.061
1.37	1.037	5.37	4.066	9.37	7.094	13.37	10.123	17.37	13.152
1.50	1.136	5.50	4.164	9.50	7.193	13.50	10.221	17.50	13.250
1.62	1.227	5.62	4.255	9.62	7.284	13.62	10.312	17.62	13.341
1.75	1.325	5.75	4.354	9.75	7.382	13.75	10.411	17.75	13.439
1.87	1.416	5.87	4.444	9.87	7.473	13.87	10.502	17.87	13.530
2.00	1.514	6.00	4.543	10.00	7.571	14.00	10.600	18.00	13.629
2.12	1.605	6.12	4.634	10.12	7.662	14.12	10.691	18.12	13.719
2.25	1.704	6.25	4.732	10.25	7.761	14.25	10.789	18.25	13.818
2.37	1.794	6.37	4.823	10.37	7.852	14.37	10.880	18.37	13.909
2.50	1.893	6.50	4.921	10.50	7.950	14.50	10.979	18.50	14.007
2.62	1.984	6.62	5.012	10.62	8.041	14.62	11.069	18.62	14.098
2.75	2.082	6.75	5.111	10.75	8.139	14.75	11.168	18.75	14.196
2.87	2.173	6.87	5.202	10.87	8.230	14.87	11.259	18.87	14.287
3.00	2.271	7.00	5.300	11.00	8.329	15.00	11.357	19.00	14.386
3.12	2.362	7.12	5.391	11.12	8.419	15.12	11.448	19.12	14.477
3.25	2.461	7.25	5.489	11.25	8.518	15.25	11.546	19.25	14.575
3.37	2.552	7.37	5.580	11.37	8.609	15.37	11.637	19.37	14.666
3.50	2.650	7.50	5.679	11.50	8.707	15.50	11.736	19.50	14.764
3.62	2.741	7.62	5.769	11.62	8.798	15.62	11.827	19.62	14.855
3.75	2.839	7.75	5.868	11.75	8.896	15.75	11.925	19.75	14.954
3.87	2.930	7.87	5.959	11.87	8.987	15.87	12.016	19.87	15.044
4.00	3.029	8.00	6.057	12.00	9.086	16.00	12.114	20.00	15.143

The second column (compensation) gives the amount of power or curve in 1.7 index material necessary to achieve the power in the first column. The basis for the first column is traditionally 1.530 index.

The compensation factor is calculated by the following formula:

$$\frac{1.530 - 1}{1.700 - 1} = 0.757142857$$

For example, what power must you grind in 1.7 index material if the requested prescription power is −9.00?

$$0.757142857 \times -9 = -6.81428571$$

F. Thickness Difference for Sharp-Edged Prisms, 1.498 Index

Prism Amount	\multicolumn{12}{c}{Prism Length or Distance between Calipering Points}
	38	40	42	44	46	48	50	52	54	56	58	60
0.50	0.38	0.40	0.42	0.44	0.46	0.48	0.50	0.52	0.54	0.56	0.58	0.60
1.00	0.76	0.80	0.84	0.88	0.92	0.96	1.00	1.04	1.08	1.12	1.16	1.20
1.50	1.14	1.20	1.27	1.33	1.39	1.45	1.51	1.57	1.63	1.69	1.75	1.81
2.00	1.53	1.61	1.69	1.77	1.85	1.93	2.01	2.09	2.17	2.25	2.33	2.41
2.50	1.91	2.01	2.11	2.21	2.31	2.41	2.51	2.61	2.71	2.81	2.91	3.01
3.00	2.29	2.41	2.53	2.65	2.77	2.89	3.01	3.13	3.25	3.37	3.49	3.61
3.50	2.67	2.81	2.95	3.09	3.23	3.37	3.51	3.65	3.80	3.94	4.08	4.22
4.00	3.05	3.21	3.37	3.53	3.69	3.86	4.02	4.18	4.34	4.50	4.66	4.82
4.50	3.43	3.61	3.80	3.98	4.16	4.34	4.52	4.70	4.88	5.06	5.24	5.42
5.00	3.82	4.02	4.22	4.42	4.62	4.82	5.02	5.22	5.42	5.62	5.82	6.02
5.50	4.20	4.42	4.64	4.86	5.08	5.30	5.52	5.74	5.96	6.18	6.41	6.63
6.00	4.58	4.82	5.06	5.30	5.54	5.78	6.02	6.27	6.51	6.75	6.99	7.23
6.50	4.96	5.22	5.48	5.74	6.00	6.27	6.53	6.79	7.05	7.31	7.57	7.83
7.00	5.34	5.62	5.90	6.18	6.47	6.75	7.03	7.31	7.59	7.87	8.15	8.43
7.50	5.72	6.02	6.33	6.63	6.93	7.23	7.53	7.83	8.13	8.43	8.73	9.04
8.00	6.10	6.43	6.75	7.07	7.39	7.71	8.03	8.35	8.67	9.00	9.32	9.64
8.50	6.49	6.83	7.17	7.51	7.85	8.19	8.53	8.88	9.22	9.56	9.90	10.24
9.00	6.87	7.23	7.59	7.95	8.31	8.67	9.04	9.40	9.76	10.12	10.48	10.84
9.50	7.25	7.63	8.01	8.39	8.78	9.16	9.54	9.92	10.30	10.68	11.06	11.45
10.00	7.63	8.03	8.43	8.84	9.24	9.64	10.04	10.44	10.84	11.24	11.65	12.05

$$d = \frac{L\Delta}{\mu - 1}$$

The difference in thickness is equal to the length of the prism in meters times the amount of prism, divided by the index of refraction minus one. (The length of the prism is the distance between calipering points.) For example, What is the thickness difference at calipering points 48mm apart for a 4.00D prism?

$$d = \frac{L\Delta}{\mu - 1}$$

$$d = \frac{(0.48)(4)}{1.498 - 1}$$

$$d = 3.86$$

G. Thickness Difference for Sharp-Edged Prisms, 1.523 Index

Prism Amount	Prism Length or Distance between Calipering Points											
	38	40	42	44	46	48	50	52	54	56	58	60
0.50	0.36	0.38	0.40	0.42	0.44	0.46	0.48	0.50	0.52	0.54	0.56	0.57
1.00	0.73	0.76	0.80	0.84	0.88	0.92	0.96	0.99	1.03	1.07	1.11	1.15
1.50	1.09	1.15	1.20	1.26	1.32	1.38	1.43	1.49	1.55	1.61	1.66	1.72
2.00	1.45	1.53	1.61	1.68	1.76	1.84	1.91	1.99	2.07	2.14	2.22	2.29
2.50	1.82	1.91	2.01	2.10	2.20	2.29	2.39	2.49	2.58	2.68	2.77	2.87
3.00	2.18	2.29	2.41	2.52	2.64	2.75	2.87	2.98	3.10	3.21	3.33	3.44
3.50	2.54	2.68	2.81	2.94	3.08	3.21	3.35	3.48	3.61	3.75	3.88	4.02
4.00	2.91	3.06	3.21	3.37	3.52	3.67	3.82	3.98	4.13	4.28	4.44	4.59
4.50	3.27	3.44	3.61	3.79	3.96	4.13	4.30	4.47	4.65	4.82	4.99	5.16
5.00	3.63	3.82	4.02	4.21	4.40	4.59	4.78	4.97	5.16	5.35	5.54	5.74
5.50	4.00	4.21	4.42	4.63	4.84	5.05	5.26	5.47	5.68	5.89	6.10	6.31
6.00	4.36	4.59	4.82	5.05	5.28	5.51	5.74	5.96	6.20	6.43	6.65	6.88
6.50	4.72	4.97	5.22	5.47	5.72	5.97	6.21	6.46	6.71	6.96	7.21	7.46
7.00	5.09	5.35	5.62	5.89	6.16	6.42	6.69	6.96	7.23	7.50	7.76	8.03
7.50	5.45	5.74	6.02	6.31	6.60	6.88	7.17	7.46	7.74	8.03	8.32	8.60
8.00	5.81	6.12	6.42	6.73	7.04	7.34	7.65	7.95	8.26	8.57	8.87	9.18
8.50	6.18	6.50	6.83	7.15	7.48	7.80	8.13	8.45	8.78	9.10	9.43	9.75
9.00	6.54	6.88	7.23	7.57	7.92	8.26	8.60	8.95	9.29	9.64	9.98	10.33
9.50	6.90	7.27	7.63	8.00	8.36	8.72	9.08	9.45	9.81	10.17	10.54	10.90
10.00	7.27	7.65	8.03	8.41	8.80	9.18	9.56	9.94	10.33	10.71	11.09	11.47

$$d = \frac{L\Delta}{\mu - 1}$$

The difference in thickness is equal to the length of the prism in meters times the amount of prism, divided by the index of refraction minus one. (The length of the prism is the distance between calipering points.) For example, What is the thickness difference at calipering points 48mm apart for a 4.00D prism?

$$d = \frac{L\Delta}{\mu - 1}$$

$$d = \frac{(0.48)(4)}{1.523 - 1}$$

$$d = 3.67$$

H. Resultant Prism of Two Prisms Crossed at 90 Degrees

Base In or Base Out

		0.25	0.50	0.75	1.00	1.25	1.50	1.75	2.00	2.25	2.50	
Base	0.25	0.35	0.56	0.79	1.03	1.27	1.52	1.77	2.02	2.26	2.51	Amount
		45	27	18	14	11	9	8	7	6	6	Axis
Up	0.50	0.56	0.71	0.90	1.12	1.35	1.58	1.82	2.06	2.30	2.55	
or		63	45	34	27	22	18	16	14	13	11	
Base	0.75	0.79	0.90	1.06	1.25	1.46	1.68	1.90	2.14	2.37	2.61	
Down		72	56	45	37	31	27	23	21	18	17	
	1.00	1.03	1.12	1.25	1.41	1.60	1.80	2.02	2.24	2.46	2.69	
		76	63	53	45	39	34	30	27	24	22	
	1.25	1.27	1.35	1.46	1.60	1.77	1.95	2.15	2.36	2.57	2.80	
		79	68	59	51	45	40	36	32	29	27	
	1.50	1.52	1.58	1.68	1.80	1.95	2.12	2.30	2.50	2.70	2.92	
		81	72	63	56	50	45	41	37	34	31	
	1.75	1.77	1.82	1.90	2.02	2.15	2.30	2.47	2.66	2.85	3.05	
		82	74	67	60	54	49	45	41	38	35	
	2.00	2.02	2.06	2.14	2.24	2.36	2.50	2.66	2.83	3.01	3.20	
		83	76	69	63	58	53	49	45	42	39	
	2.25	2.26	2.30	2.37	2.46	2.57	2.70	2.85	3.01	3.18	3.36	
		84	77	72	66	61	56	52	48	45	42	
	2.50	2.51	2.55	2.61	2.69	2.80	2.92	3.05	3.20	3.36	3.54	
		84	79	73	68	63	59	55	51	48	45	
	2.75	2.76	2.80	2.85	2.93	3.02	3.13	3.26	3.40	3.55	3.72	
		85	80	75	70	66	61	58	54	51	48	
	3.00	3.01	3.04	3.09	3.16	3.25	3.35	3.47	3.61	3.75	3.91	
		85	81	76	72	67	63	60	56	53	50	
	3.25	3.26	3.29	3.34	3.40	3.48	3.58	3.69	3.82	3.95	4.10	
		86	81	77	73	69	65	62	58	55	52	
	3.50	3.51	3.54	3.58	3.64	3.72	3.81	3.91	4.03	4.16	4.30	
		86	82	78	74	70	67	63	60	57	54	
	3.75	3.76	3.78	3.82	3.88	3.95	4.04	4.14	4.25	4.37	4.51	
		86	82	79	75	72	68	65	62	59	56	
	4.00	4.01	4.03	4.07	4.12	4.19	4.27	4.37	4.47	4.59	4.72	
		86	83	79	76	73	69	66	63	61	58	
	4.25	4.26	4.28	4.32	4.37	4.43	4.51	4.60	4.70	4.81	4.93	
		87	83	80	77	74	71	68	65	62	60	
	4.50	4.51	4.53	4.56	4.61	4.67	4.74	4.83	4.92	5.03	5.15	
		87	84	81	77	74	72	69	66	63	61	
	4.75	4.76	4.78	4.81	4.85	4.91	4.98	5.06	5.15	5.26	5.37	
		87	84	81	78	75	72	70	67	65	62	
	5.00	5.01	5.02	5.06	5.10	5.15	5.22	5.30	5.39	5.48	5.59	
		87	84	81	79	76	73	71	68	66	63	

$$R = \sqrt{P_1^2 + P_2^2}$$

The resultant prism equals the square root of the first prism squared plus the second prism squared.

I. Resultant Prism of Two Prisms Crossed at 90 Degrees
Base In or Base Out

		2.75	3.00	3.25	3.50	3.75	4.00	4.25	4.50	4.75	5.00	
Base	0.25	2.76	3.01	3.26	3.51	3.76	4.01	4.26	4.51	4.76	5.01	Amount
		5	5	4	4	4	4	3	3	3	3	Axis
Up	0.50	2.80	3.04	3.29	3.54	3.78	4.03	4.28	4.53	4.78	5.02	
or		10	9	9	8	8	7	7	6	6	6	
Base	0.75	2.85	3.09	3.34	3.58	3.82	4.07	4.32	4.56	4.81	5.06	
Down		15	14	13	12	11	11	10	9	9	9	
	1.00	2.93	3.16	3.40	3.64	3.88	4.12	4.37	4.61	4.85	5.10	
		20	18	17	16	15	14	13	13	12	11	
	1.25	3.02	3.25	3.48	3.72	3.95	4.19	4.43	4.67	4.91	5.15	
		24	23	21	20	18	17	16	16	15	14	
	1.50	3.13	3.35	3.58	3.81	4.04	4.27	4.51	4.74	4.98	5.22	
		29	27	25	23	22	21	19	18	18	17	
	1.75	3.26	3.47	3.69	3.91	4.14	4.37	4.60	4.83	5.06	5.30	
		32	30	28	27	25	24	22	21	20	19	
	2.00	3.40	3.61	3.82	4.03	4.25	4.47	4.70	4.92	5.15	5.39	
		36	34	32	30	28	27	25	24	23	22	
	2.25	3.55	3.75	3.95	4.16	4.37	4.59	4.81	5.03	5.26	5.48	
		39	37	35	33	31	29	28	27	25	24	
	2.50	3.72	3.91	4.10	4.30	4.51	4.72	4.93	5.15	5.37	5.59	
		42	40	38	36	34	32	30	29	28	27	
	2.75	3.89	4.07	4.26	4.45	4.65	4.85	5.06	5.27	5.49	5.71	
		45	43	40	38	36	35	33	31	30	29	
	3.00	4.07	4.24	4.42	4.61	4.80	5.00	5.20	5.41	5.62	5.83	
		47	45	43	41	39	37	35	34	32	31	
	3.25	4.26	4.42	4.60	4.78	4.96	5.15	5.35	5.55	5.76	5.96	
		50	47	45	43	41	39	37	36	34	33	
	3.50	4.45	4.61	4.78	4.95	5.13	5.32	5.51	5.70	5.90	6.10	
		52	49	47	45	43	41	39	38	36	35	
	3.75	4.65	4.80	4.96	5.13	5.30	5.48	5.67	5.86	6.05	6.25	
		54	51	49	47	45	43	41	40	38	37	
	4.00	4.85	5.00	5.15	5.32	5.48	5.66	5.84	6.02	6.21	6.40	
		55	53	51	49	47	45	43	42	40	39	
	4.25	5.06	5.20	5.35	5.51	5.67	5.84	6.01	6.19	6.37	6.56	
		57	55	53	51	49	47	45	43	42	40	
	4.50	5.27	5.41	5.55	5.70	5.86	6.02	6.19	6.36	6.54	6.73	
		59	56	54	52	50	48	47	45	43	42	
	4.75	5.49	5.62	5.76	5.90	6.05	6.21	6.37	6.54	6.72	6.90	
		60	58	56	54	52	50	48	47	45	44	
	5.00	5.71	5.83	5.96	6.10	6.25	6.40	6.56	6.73	6.90	7.07	
		61	59	57	55	53	51	50	48	46	45	

$$\tan A = \frac{P_1}{P_2}$$

The tangent of the angle is equal to the prism up or prism down divided by the prism in or prism out. This will give you the amount the axis deviates from the 180 degree line.

J.   Diopters to Radius in Millimeters, 1.530

Diop.	Rad.	Diop.	Rad.	Diop.	Rad.	Diop.	Rad.	Diop.	Rad.
0.12	4416.67	4.12	128.64	8.12	65.27	12.12	43.73	16.12	32.88
0.25	2120.00	4.25	124.71	8.25	64.24	12.25	43.27	16.25	32.62
0.37	1432.43	4.37	121.28	8.37	63.32	12.37	42.85	16.37	32.38
0.50	1060.00	4.50	117.78	8.50	62.35	12.50	42.40	16.50	32.12
0.62	854.84	4.62	114.72	8.62	61.48	12.62	42.00	16.62	31.89
0.75	706.67	4.75	111.58	8.75	60.57	12.75	41.57	16.75	31.64
0.87	609.20	4.87	108.83	8.87	59.75	12.87	41.18	16.87	31.42
1.00	530.00	5.00	106.00	9.00	58.89	13.00	40.77	17.00	31.18
1.12	473.21	5.12	103.52	9.12	58.11	13.12	40.40	17.12	30.96
1.25	424.00	5.25	100.95	9.25	57.30	13.25	40.00	17.25	30.72
1.37	386.86	5.37	98.70	9.37	56.56	13.37	39.64	17.37	30.51
1.50	353.33	5.50	96.36	9.50	55.79	13.50	39.26	17.50	30.29
1.62	327.16	5.62	94.31	9.62	55.09	13.62	38.91	17.62	30.08
1.75	302.86	5.75	92.17	9.75	54.36	13.75	38.55	17.75	29.86
1.87	283.42	5.87	90.29	9.87	53.70	13.87	38.21	17.87	29.66
2.00	265.00	6.00	88.33	10.00	53.00	14.00	37.86	18.00	29.44
2.12	250.00	6.12	86.60	10.12	52.37	14.12	37.54	18.12	29.25
2.25	235.56	6.25	84.80	10.25	51.71	14.25	37.19	18.25	29.04
2.37	223.63	6.37	83.20	10.37	51.11	14.37	36.88	18.37	28.85
2.50	212.00	6.50	81.54	10.50	50.48	14.50	36.55	18.50	28.65
2.62	202.29	6.62	80.06	10.62	49.91	14.62	36.25	18.62	28.46
2.75	192.73	6.75	78.52	10.75	49.30	14.75	35.93	18.75	28.27
2.87	184.67	6.87	77.15	10.87	48.76	14.87	35.64	18.87	28.09
3.00	176.67	7.00	75.71	11.00	48.18	15.00	35.33	19.00	27.89
3.12	169.87	7.12	74.44	11.12	47.66	15.12	35.05	19.12	27.72
3.25	163.08	7.25	73.10	11.25	47.11	15.25	34.75	19.25	27.53
3.37	157.27	7.37	71.91	11.37	46.61	15.37	34.48	19.37	27.36
3.50	151.43	7.50	70.67	11.50	46.09	15.50	34.19	19.50	27.18
3.62	146.41	7.62	69.55	11.62	45.61	15.62	33.93	19.62	27.01
3.75	141.33	7.75	68.39	11.75	45.11	15.75	33.65	19.75	26.84
3.87	136.95	7.87	67.34	11.87	44.65	15.87	33.40	19.87	26.67
4.00	132.50	8.00	66.25	12.00	44.17	16.00	33.13	20.00	26.50

The second column (radius) gives the equivalent radius of curvature in millimeters of the first column's diopter value. The radius of curvature is calculated using the following formula:

$$R = \frac{\mu - 1}{\text{Diopter}}$$

The radius of curvature in meters is equal to the index of refraction minus one, divided by the diopter value. For example, what is the radius of curvature of 5.00D?

$$R = \frac{1.530 - 1}{5}$$

$$R = \quad 0.106 \text{ meters, or } 106mm$$

APPENDIX I

Measuring Employee Productivity

The implementation of an accurate method to measure employee productivity is the first step to an improved profit margin. Surfaces per worker hour is the traditional way to measure surface shop productivity. However, this method is comparatively less successful in the finish shop. A newer alternative considers the shop as a unit, using as its basis the number of outgoing prescriptions per person—finish and surface shop combined. This is nothing more than another way of looking at surfaces per worker hour. The problem is that surfaces per worker hour is an irrelevant statistic.

Since statistics cannot pay bills, we should base our productivity on what does—money. Surfaces per worker *dollar* is a better comparison. For example, a surface shop composed of one experienced apprentice at $5.00 per hour and two machine operators at $3.50 per hour generates 120 worker hours per week. A surface shop composed of one journeyman at $8.00 per hour and one experienced apprentice at $5.00 per hour generates only 80 worker hours per week. The first shop with the three employees costs $12.00 per hour to operate, while the second shop with only two employees costs $13.00 per hour to operate. If you could get the work out with either shop, you would be farther ahead with the three-employee shop for several reasons, including the following:

1. It would cost less to operate.
2. You would have better coverage for vacations, illness, and other employee and employer emergencies.

The surfaces per worker hour would not look very good, but the surfaces per worker dollar would be superior. After all, are we not primarily concerned with the bottom-line dollar; I suggest we replace our antiquated system of surfaces per worker hour with the more fundamentally sound surfaces per worker dollar.

Do not misconstrue this simplistic example as suggesting the demise of the journeyman. The point is to consider both your costs and needs. Your employee's cost to you is far greater than simply their salary. Do not forget to add on the costs of all benefits such as insurance, vacation pay, profit sharing, and so forth. This is why two part-time employees at twenty hours each and no company benefits are far less expensive than one full-time employee with company benefits at the same base salary.

I do not mean to imply that we should turn to the generally least-caring, least-costly part-time help we can find. We must, however not lose sight of the tremendous technological advances in our industry. The advent of inexpensive computers and highly automated lens-fabricating machinery has changed dramatically the ratio of top-shelf journeymen to machine operators needed to properly operate a lab. Obviously, you need some highly skilled journeymen to insure the proper operation of the lab. At the same time, however, we must be careful to use the journeymen's talents to the fullest, confining their work to that which cannot be done by someone of lesser ability and at a lower wage.

While surfaces per worker dollar is the easiest way to figure productivity in a production lab, even this system has its problems in the highly skilled, complete lab that does slabs, minus lenticulars, low-vision aids, and soforth. It obviously takes a good deal more time and knowledge to fabricate one of these "trick jobs" than a standard production job. Figuring productivity in this type of shop is only slightly more complicated but a good deal more accurate than for a standard job using the following method. Instead of figuring each outgoing prescription as a unit that is equal to all the other outgoing units (as in the surfaces per worker dollar system), simply consider the dollar value of the prescriptions. Instead of dividing the amount of worker dollars into the number of units, you would divide worker dollars into the dollars you bill your accounts. Since your price list should reflect both the cost of materials and the cost of production, this system will allow you to compare the easiest and most difficult of jobs on a production basis. This will give you a clear look at your profit margin based on the cost of labor only.

If your margin is already poor at this point prior to figuring the balance of your overhead, you must consider two things. Either the price list is too low, or productivity must be increased. The solution to the first is simple—raise your prices. The second is a bit more complex. Remember, productivity is not only the speed of work but also its cost. The cost of production can be lowered several ways:

1. Using more efficient machinery. This will allow you to accomplish more in less time.
2. Using more automated machinery. This will allow you to switch to the less-skilled, lower-paid employee.
3. Changing the prescription-per-employee ratio by either obtaining additional work or laying people off.

Before considering any of these options, make sure your employees are working up to their abilities. If not, you must either inspire or fire.

To summarize, the easiest way to measure productivity is by the outgoing units or surfaces per worker dollar. Simply divide the amount of money needed to get the work out (worker dollars) into the amount of outgoing units or surfaces, depending on which you are measuring. If you do work other than production, or if you want to use the most accurate method, simply replace units in this formula with your account billing amount and divide by the worker dollars. This will give you the dollars of outgoing prescription per dollar of employee overhead, that is, productivity.

APPENDIX II
Account Relations

Ours is a very specialized and rapidly changing profession. Ophthalmologists, optometrists, and opticians keep busy enough staying up to date in their own fields without trying to master everyone elses'. It is not the lab's place to question the method of obtaining or the relevance of a prescription. However, with our up-to-the-minute knowledge of our field, we may have a new way to better fabricate a prescription. New lenses, frames, and ideas abound in our profession.

Keep informed those accounts who appreciate your knowledge. Do not hesitate to make suggestions or ask questions. We all make mistakes. Perhaps that prescription that looks ridiculous was simply written incorrectly. You could save everyone time and money by making a simply inquiry. A good lab should be in contact with the account, making relevant suggestions and inquiries. Saying the prescription cannot be done is of no help to the account without suggesting an alternative. If they knew the prescription could not or should not be done, they would not have sent it to begin with. Therefore, the odds are they have no idea what the best solution or alternative is.

Always be ready with solutions—not problems. Avoid using the word *cannot*. The desire to obtain accounts coupled with the love of challenge is all some people need to figure out a way to fabricate a prescription. It is not a question of whether or not a prescription can be fabricated, but rather if the results are optically and aesthetically sound. If the frame size, PD, style of lens, or any combination of these or other factors makes a ridiculous prescription, do not say the prescription cannot be fabricated. Instead, point out that the prescription will not be optically or aesthetically sound and advise the account how to rectify the problem. If the account insists on the ridiculous, inform them of the extra charges they can expect because of the prescription's unusual nature. Also note on the prescription what you advised and the account's decision. You may not remember this later when the account tells you the prescription was fabricated incorrectly. Making notations is not for the purpose of arguing with an account. A lab that argues with accounts loses them. The true purpose of these notations is to establish and protect your professional integrity.

Accounts will listen and cooperate far better after you have established your knowledge and professional sincerity. We should never lose sight of the fact that a cooperative effort will best achieve the goal of bringing good vision to the patient.

APPENDIX III
Plastic Troubleshooting Guide

When you have a fabrication problem, the first and most important thing to do is narrow down the possibilities. Is the problem really occurring on *all* the lenses? Which manufacturer and base curves? On which inside curves? Spheres, cylinders, or both? What time of day or week? (For determining the condition of employees, slurry, etc.) The following troubleshooting guide lists some of the most prevalent problems and some possible solutions. It should provide an excellent starting point toward solving your problem. For further information about correct procedures, refer back to the appropriate chapter in the text.

Waves

Precoat

Applying the precoat evenly is extremely important. A very uneven coating will allow the heat from the alloy at blocking to unevenly affect the lens surface, and this could cause waves.

Blocking

Another heat-related problem would be caused if the alloy were too hot or the blocks not cold enough. The alloy would not be cooling rapidly enough and, thus, would overheat the surface of the lens.

Water trapped between the block and the lens can also cause a wave. This water could be from either poorly dried blocks or condensation from the surface of the chilled block. Condensation should be wiped off prior to blocking.

Check the block centers for wear. Worn centers will cause waves.

Generating

Heat buildup while generating could possibly wave a lens. Factors to watch include proper coolant flow, adequate cooling time prior to generating, and as few heat-building cuts as possible.

The other possible problem at the generator is an inside curve wave (as opposed to the blocked side wave that we have discussed up to now). An inside curve wave can be caused by either the lens bending while being generated or the generator slipping in curve or takeoff. A poor curve will result in these cases. If if is not noticed during fining or polishing, an inside curve wave can result.

Fining and Polishing

If the lens is not adequately beveled, small pieces of plastic or precoat can work their way between the lens and tool, creating a wave. Any contamination in the slurry can react in the same manner.

Fining pads must be put on smoothly. A pad with a crease or bump in it can cause a wave. It would be wise to use a pad press. To avoid generator-created problems, make sure all the generator marks have been removed and the entire surface has been completely fined and polished out.

Carefully check the fit between the block centers and the cylinder machine pins. Excessive wear of either can cause enough play to create waves.

Another area of possible concern is the machine itself. Incorrect or varying pressure can cause waves. Sloppy bearings or loose parts in general can be a problem. Make sure all parts have freedom of movement throughout their cycle, without sloppy play. With the machine off, grab both the pin and table assemblies and attempt to move them back and forth. While you are doing this, feel and listen for play. Consult the manufacturer's manual for repairs and other possible problem areas.

Deblocking

If you melt the lenses off, make sure the water is not too hot. There is no reason for the temperature to be over 125°F. This is another case where excessive heat could wave the lens.

A wave that was created by heat can possibly be removed by heat. If the wave is not too bad, the oven may remove it. You may also wish to consider a cause of waves not related to fabrication. The quality of the lens used can greatly affect the results. Did the lens have a front side wave from the manufacturer? How about internal striae from manufacturing? Was the lens properly cured? These are but a few of the possible causes of waved lenses. Waves can be elusive. If you go through this list carefully, by the process of elimination you will probably find the cause of your problem. Many other surface problems, like "orange peel," are created and can be cured in the same manner as a waved lens.

Scratches

Markup

Overly aggressive markup or something on the marking device can scratch a lens. The lens should be marked gently. There is no reason to bear down with the marking pencil.

Precoat

You cannot expect a lens to make it through the shop free of scratches unless it has been precoated adequately. Precoat must be applied evenly and completely across the lens surface. Care should also be taken so the applicator does not contain any foreign bodies that could scratch the lens. If the precoat is being applied by an air gun, make sure the air line is filtered. The filter will trap rust or other foreign bodies to help prevent scratches.

Blocking

When the lens is placed on the blocking mold, do not allow the lens to slide. If the lens slides against the mold, the precoat could tear and the lens could become scratched.

Generating

Do not spin the generator chucking ring against the lens; this could tear the precoat and scratch the lens.

When generating both glass and plastic with the same generator, it is important to keep cut glass away from plastic lenses. Keep both the cutting chamber and coolant clean of excessive glass contamination.

Fining and Polishing

Care must be taken to protect both sides of the lens. Do not carelessly slide the calipers across the lens surfaces. Use ball-tipped calipers on plastic lenses. Make sure deep scratches are fined out on the minus side. Do not expect the polisher to remove more scratches than it can.

Carefully wash clean both the lens and tool before going to the polisher. This should keep most of the scratch-producing, finer contaminants out of the polish. Keep a good bevel on the lens. Small particles of loose plastic can scratch either surface.

If you use a very coarse fining pad, or if the slurry gets too contaminated, the slurry should be changed.

Deblocking and Cleaning

When melting the lens off, do not slide it. When the alloy is adequately melted the lens will lift off. Do not knock the lens off against a sharp surface. Avoid excessive rubbing when carefully cleaning the lens. Consult the chapter on cleaning for the correct procedure.

Assuming the lens has come from the manufacturer free of scratches, scratches are caused by sloppy work habits. Keep the shop, equipment, and employees clean. Even a factor such as how the shop is laid out can affect scratching. Powder from glass, glass cylinder machines, grinders, tool cutters, etc., can fill the air with scratch-producing agents. Keep a good, complete barrier between these agents and your plastic operation. However, the most important element is a caring employee.

Gray

Generating

An improperly cut curve on the generator can create an eventual gray area if not caught on the finer.

Fining and Polishing

The most obvious cause of gray is incomplete fining or polishing. Make certain all the generator marks are fined out. This will insure a generator-to-tool curve match and will eliminate generator-induced gray.

Make sure you are using the correct tool and that its curve has been cut correctly.

Incorrect pad pattern or thickness match-ups can cause gray.

There are several possible polish-oriented problems. There should be an adequate flow of polish, and it should not be too warm. The Baumé of the polish can be checked to determine if it is broken down too much. Machine problems or limitations can also cause gray. Incorrect or varying pressure can create gray. Also, be concerned with the length of the machine stroke. The lens may be too large to be properly fined and polished in a normal position. If this is the case, offset the lens to both sides and then to the center to obtain the needed coverage. If you are not using on-center blocking, the lens should be centered on the tool to be properly fined and polished.

If you look at these basic causes of gray, you will notice that they all seem to have one thing in common: poor work habits stand out as the basic cause. This is the case whether you are talking about inattentive processing or poor machine maintenance. Gray should be an easy problem to eliminate.

Prism

Shop Slip

The prism calculations and/or computer entries should be carefully checked.

Markup

Check the direction of the prism and the placement of the prism base arrow. Are the prism rings marked at the base or apex?

Blocking

The accuracy of the blocker should be checked if it is the type that blocks in the prism. If it is not, make sure you are not accidentally inducing prism. Are the blocks clean of alloy? After blocking, is the excess alloy removed to avoid prism from generator chucking?

Generating

If you are constantly obtaining the same amount of prism, as measured with a caliper, the generator could be at fault. The generator manual should be consulted for the proper adjustment. If you make a habit of calipering the lenses off the generator, the finer can correct most prism problems. You can also notice if the amount is usually about the same and, thus, correct the generator problem. Correct chucking will also help eliminate prism. Refer to the text and your generator manual for the correct procedure.

Inspect the generator chuck. If there is any alloy or any other foreign body in it, prism will result. Obviously, the correct selection of the generator ring and its proper placement on the lens are very important.

Fining and Polishing

Unequal pressure across the lens is the major cause of prism during fining and polishing. The unequal pressure can come from two basic areas. First, if the lens is not correctly centered, unequal pressure will create prism. The second source of unequal pressure is the machine itself. Poor or unequal pressure can be the result of several machine problems; everything from air line variations and stroke problems to baffle tightness can cause problems. Consult your operator's manual for repairs and other possible problem areas.

The chapter on removing prism describes how to rectify your problem once it exists. However, it is best to eliminate the need to remove the prism. There are not too many places where prism can be induced. You should work to eliminate prism rather than becoming an expert at removing it from the lens.

Power

Shop Slip

All calculations should be checked for accuracy. The accuracy of the computer entires should also be checked. Re-sag the lens to determine if the front curve has been altered in processing.

Generating

If an incorrect curve is cut on the generator and incorrectly fined, a power error could result. Is the correct shop slip with the lens?

Incorrect generator takeoff can create problems. Too thick or too thin a lens will alter the power.

Fining and Polishing

Incorrect or unmatched curves between the generator and the cylinder machines can change the power. Check the tool for curve accuracy, and make sure you are using the correct tool.

Check the power across the entire surface of the lens. A wave can cause localized power errors. (Refer to the troubleshooting section on waves.) Double-check the quality of the lens manufacturer. Look for errors in packing, poor curing, or a bad front curve. Check the plastic and pad compensations, whether they be at layout or in the tool. The reasons for power errors are relatively few and should be easy to find.

FIGURES

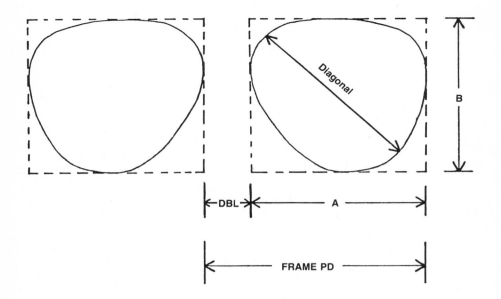

Figure 1. This is a diagram of the
standard boxing system, with one
exception: ED from the standard
boxing system has been replaced
by *diagonal*. The ED is not repre-
sentative of the actual size of the
finished lenses. Plus-powered lens
calculations based on an ED will
create much too thick a lens. Thickness problems can be minimized by
substituting the longest diagonal
measurement for the ED.

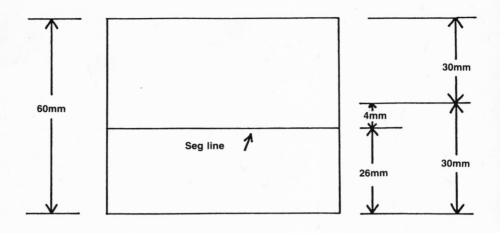

Figure 2. Executive-style segment
height.

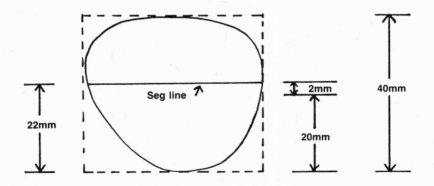

Figure 3. Determining segment
height.

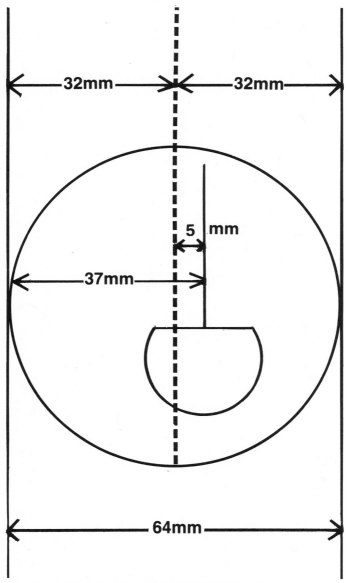

Figure 4. Flat top multifocal segment placement.

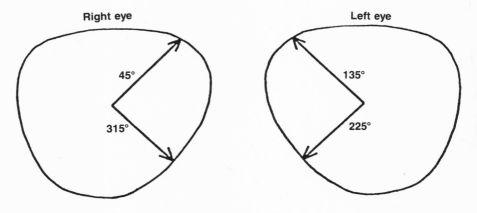

Figure 5. Determining prism axis.

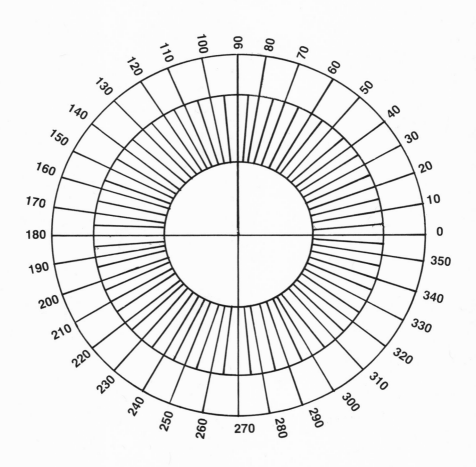

Figure 6. 360-degree protractor.

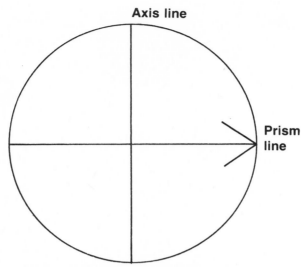

Figure 7. Single-vision lens mark-up.

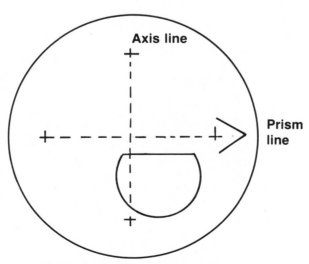

Figure 8. Multifocal lens markup.

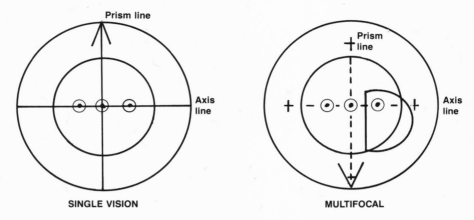

Figure 9. Alignment of lens on block.

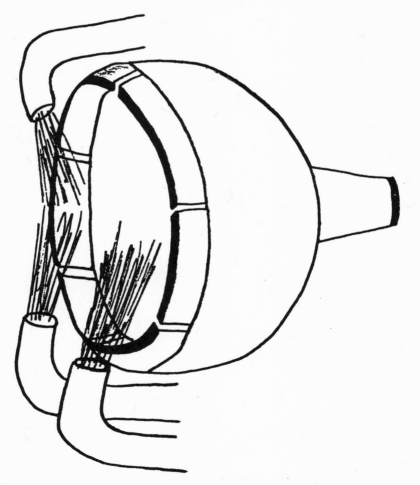

Figure 10. One of the recommended manifold spout arrangements.

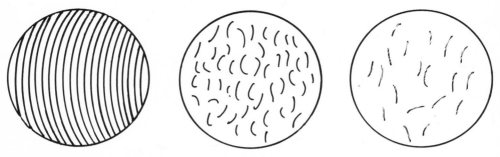

Figure 11. Generator marks (left), first fine marks (center), and second fine marks (right).

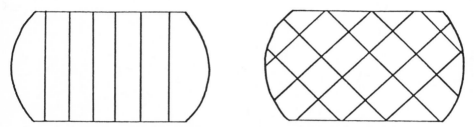

Figure 12. Vertical (left) and diagonal (right) scoring.

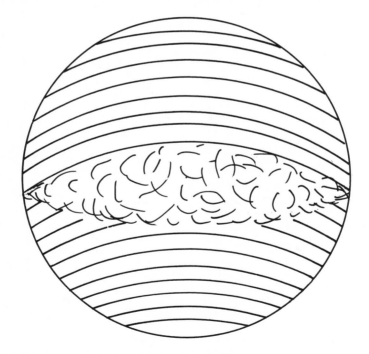

Figure 13. A lens with an incorrect generator curve discovered on the finer.

Figure 14. Calipering points.

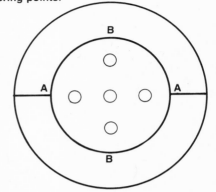

Sphere without prism: All calipering points A should be the same thickness.

Cylinder without prism: Calipering points A should be the same thickness. Calipering points B should be the same thickness, but different than points A.

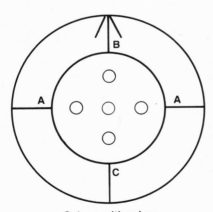

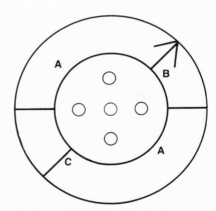

Sphere with prism

Cylinder with prism

Calipering points A should be the same thickness. The thickness difference between calipering points B and C should be the amount of prism. Points A are always 90 degrees opposite the prism line.

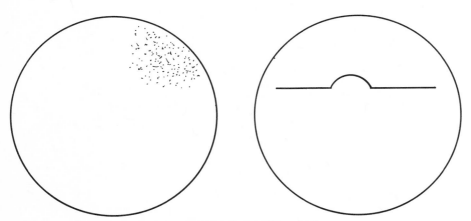

Figure 15. Lens inspection. Left: When light floods an incompletely polished lens, the gray areas will not reflect the light brightly and may appear speckled. Right: Tip a lens under a light source to form a straight line, slowly crossing the lens. If the line bends abruptly, the surface is waved.

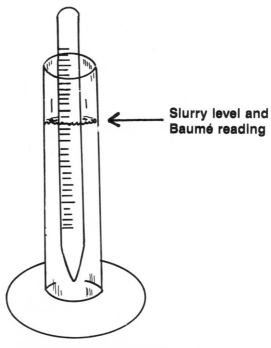

← Slurry level and Baumé reading

Figure 16. Taking a Baumé reading.

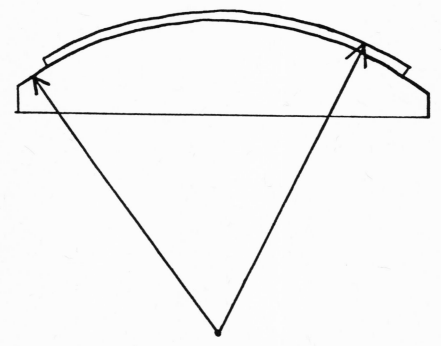

Figure 17. The radius of curvature of a padded and unpadded tool.

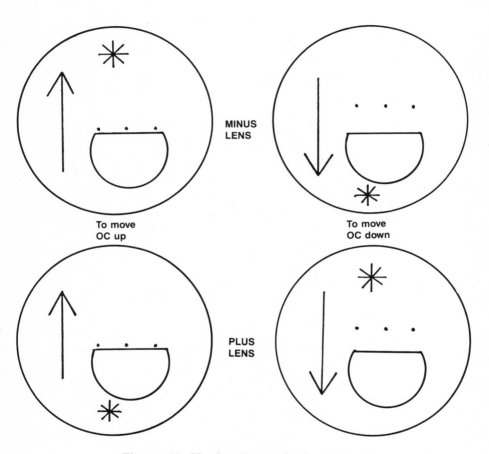

MINUS LENS

To move OC up

To move OC down

PLUS LENS

Figure 18. Moving the optical center.

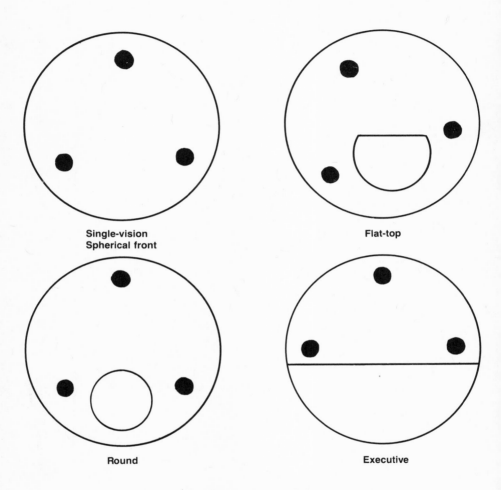

Figure 19. Spacer disk placement.

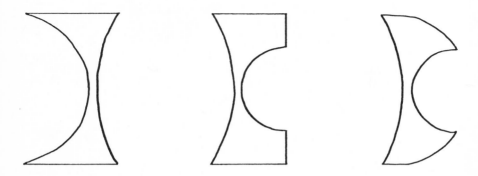

Figure 20. High minus lens treatments: double concave (left), myodisc (center), and minus lenticular (right).

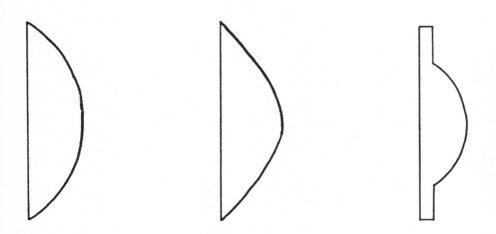

Figure 21. High plus lens treatments: spheric front (left), aspheric front (center), and aspheric lenticular front (right).

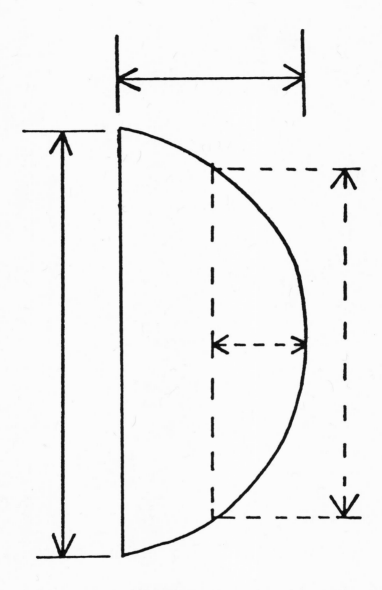

Figure 22. The relationship between the diameter and thickness of a plus lens.

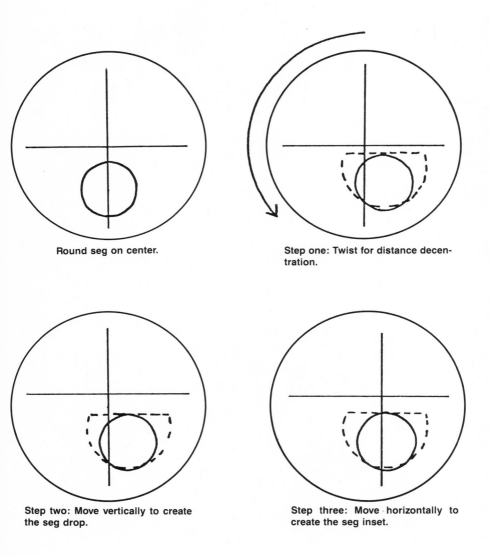

Round seg on center.

Step one: Twist for distance decentration.

Step two: Move vertically to create
the seg drop.

Step three: Move horizontally to
create the seg inset.

Figure 23. Round and blended segment markup.

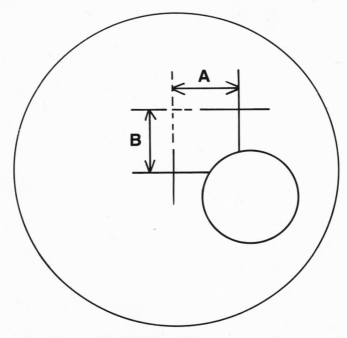

Figure 24. Compound prism markup. A is the amount the blocking center must be moved for horizontal on-center blocking. B is the amount the blocking center must be moved for vertical on-center blocking. The compound prism created by A and B will allow on-center blocking.